W9-CVT-999

DATE DUE

G. W. KORTING

Diseases of the Skin in Children and Adolescents

Diseases of the
Skin in Children and Adolescents

A Color Atlas

by

Professor G. W. KORTING, M. D.

Director, Department of Dermatology University Hospital, Mainz, Germany

American Edition Translated and Adapted

by

WILLIAM CURTH, M. D.

Associate in Dermatology (Retired), College of Physicians and Surgeons,
Columbia University; Assistant Clinical Professor, New York Medical College

and

HELEN OLLENDORFF CURTH, M. D.

Assistant Clinical Professor of Dermatology (Retired), Special Lecturer in
Dermatology, College of Physicians and Surgeons, Columbia University

With 398 figures, of which 390 are multicolored

W. B. SAUNDERS COMPANY
PHILADELPHIA · LONDON · TORONTO

Preface

The idea of pediatric dermatology is neither new nor original, as is evident from passing contributions in both older and more recent handbooks of dermatology and pediatrics, and not least of all from related monographs such as that by BRANDWEINER (1910), the famous atlas by FINKELSTEIN, GALEWSKY, and HALBERSTÄDTER, and *Pediatric Dermatology* by PERLMAN. Nevertheless, it seems necessary, in view of the emphatically gerontologic or geriatric orientation in medicine, to indicate in new monographic form that a child does not simply represent a miniature adult form, but shows basic morphologic and functional differences which apply in particular to the skin. Such dermatologic differences are found not only in the longer life of epidermal cells in childhood, but also in the higher elasticity of the tissue, and even clinically in a special disposition toward rash or tendency toward exudation or bulla formation. In addition, the apocrine glands become active mostly at the time of puberty. More important, however, are the characteristic courses of a few dermatoses in childhood, and even diagnostic dermatologic pictures, as for example, aphthous stomatitis, "juvenile warts," and mycoses of the hairy portion of the head. In contrast, it cannot be denied that certain other common skin diseases occur predominantly (though not exclusively) at older ages. This awareness of the need for taking age into account must remain viable; it therefore seemed fitting to assemble the available knowledge in the area of pediatric dermatology and to present it through text and pictures – concisely enough that even the future doctor will be able to orient himself to the knowledge at hand. In dermatology one is dependent upon acquiring and digesting precise observations. Therefore, pictures are a logical part – indeed, the fulfillment – of the textbook. Conversely, the pictorial information will frequently stimulate deeper understanding of the text material, which in this book has intentionally been kept as brief as possible. The organization of the material corresponds largely to my *Therapie der Hautkrankheiten*, to which questions pertaining to therapy, which were all but left out here, should be referred.

For the use of the following illustrations I thank Dr. BODE, of Göttingen (Figs. 13, 14, 208, 209, 211), Dr. BOPP, of Porto Alegre (Fig. 158), Dr. FEGELER, of Munich (Figs. 129, 132), Drs. GREITHER and IPPEN, of Düsseldorf (Figs. 242, 243), Dr. LOEWENTHAL, of Johannesburg (Fig. 287), Drs. MUSGER and KRESBACH, of Graz (Figs. 218, 299), and Dr. STÜTTGEN, of Frankfurt am Main (Figs. 103, 105–107). Figure 104 was taken by my colleague, Dr. NURNBERGER, with Dr. KNEEDLER at the McKean Leprosy Colony, Chiengmai, Thailand. I thank my colleague on the faculty, Dr. KÖTTGEN, not only for the use of Figures 7, 47, 177, 206, 233, 236, 257, 258, 262, and 286, but most of all for his understanding discussion of my plan and, not least, for the referral of many children with dermatologic illnesses.

For assistance in reading the manuscript I thank my scientific assistant, Dr. GEBHARDT. The photographs were made mainly by Dr. FABER, while the typing of the manuscript was as usual in the competent hands of Mrs. G. MORITZ. To The Schattauer Publishing Company, and especially Dr. MATIS, my thanks are extended for the sympathetic understanding of the author's demanding standards, and most of all, despite high cost, for reproduction of the color photographs.

G. W. KORTING

V

Contents

VIII

XII

1. Acute Erythemas and Exanthems

Erythema is the simplest reaction of the skin to various irritants. Reddening is caused by arteriolar or capillary hyperemia. Flat red spots of various sizes may appear in the level of the surrounding normal skin. These macules may become slightly elevated or moderately urticarial because of fluid exuded from the vessels. Erythemas are common in children, and the disposition to an erythematous reaction in infants is well known.

An *exanthem* (an *enanthem* if occurring on a mucous membrane) is characterized by many small single eruptive lesions which have developed endogenously via the blood stream, or less frequently the lymphatics or nerve impulses. The erythema may become more intense, wane and show occasional recurrences, and finally subside.

Erythroderma refers to generalized macular redness, often accompanied by swelling and scaling. At later stages of development the integument may be involved from head to foot. Erythroderma frequently occurs secondary to another dermatosis (eczema, psoriasis vulgaris, lichen planus, and so forth). Primary erythroderma may appear on previously normal skin as a result of reticuloendothelioses and other causes. Regardless of its origin, if an erythroderma has been present for some time, the patient shows certain accompanying pathologic signs such as chills, fever, an increased basal metabolic rate, cutaneous loss of fluid, and a disposition to hypergammaglobulinemia. In children, certain gastrointestinal manifestations may also be observed.

In infants *desquamative erythroderma* (LEINER) represents the most severe form of seborrheic eczema. *Congenital ichthyosiform erythroderma* (BROCQ), showing occasional bullous lesions, represents the inflammatory form of ichthyosis congenita. Of further interest in this age group is the erythroderma of pityriasis rubra pilaris and *erythema scarlatiniforme desquamativum recidivans* which is caused by infections or intolerance to drugs such as mercury. Recurrent attacks are also characteristic.

Toxic erythema of the newborn

Multiple erythematous lesions may appear on the trunk or extremities as early as the second or third day of life. For the most part the lesions are urticarial. They may also be morbilliform or lichenoid. At later stages they may become confluent. As a rule, the eruption disappears after a few days with no complications. Most pediatricians consider this form of erythroderma a postnatal reaction to the change of environment of the newborn.

Chancriform pyoderma

This common dermatosis of infants is known by many names, among them dermatitis pseudosyphilitica papulosa and dermatitis ammoniacalis. This common erythematous diaper rash may become aggravated, exhibiting blisters, erosions, and even firm vegetating papules. It is identical with pseudosyphilis papulosa (LIPSCHÜTZ) in an adult who is incontinent of urine or feces. Staphylococcus and yeast infections play an etiologic role in both infants and adults. Ammonia liberated in an alkaline medium is also injurious. It is therefore advisable to acidify the urine by dietary means in cases which have become resistant to therapy. In contrast to the diaper rash of acutely dyspeptic infants, in which areas of circular redness are located immediately next to the anus, erythema papulosum posterosivum does not affect the immediate circumanal region. Its location also distinguishes it from syphilitic papules.

Exanthema subitum

In 1921 VEETER and HEMPELMANN gave the name of exanthema subitum to this disorder of three days' duration. The disorder occurs in children up to two years of age. School age children are rarely affected. On the third day after sudden and high fever, an eruption appears. When the high temperature becomes normal by crises, a fleeting pink rash is seen. The rash simulates rubella or a morbilliform exanthem. Spreading centrifugally from the trunk to the extremities, the exanthem leaves the face unaffected. Appearance of the exanthem heralds the "dawn of recovery" (GLANZMANN).

Exanthema subitum exhibits a reddish hue, with no scaling or itching. The patient may, however, exhibit mild, concomitant neurologic signs, such as hypersensitivity to touch, increased tension of the fontanelles, and convulsions as a result of the high fever. The hemogram shows leukopenia and lymphomonocytosis.

Measles (rubeola)

The causative organism of this worldwide and highly contagious childhood disease belongs to the group of myxoviruses. It gains entrance to the body through the respiratory tract and the conjunctivae. After a fixed incubation period of 9 to 11 days a complex of prodromal signs, among them biphasic elevations of temperature, blepharoconjunctivitis, photophobia, rhinitis, and bronchitis, sets in. The exanthem, which appears on the thirteenth to fourteenth day, is characteristic. Sydenham has pointed out that the eruption seems to develop under the very eyes of the observer, in the form of small, faintly red spots, progressing to large dusky-red confluent areas. As in rubella, the initial lesions are located behind the ears. Because of the morbilliform nature of some of the other exanthems, the appearance of Koplik's spots (1896)*) is of great diagnostic significance. These chalky white spots are seen around the orifice of the parotid duct, opposite the premolars. They represent aggregated, superficial, epithelial necroses which may simulate elements of thrush. The latter, however, can be wiped off, leaving easily bleeding erosions. Initially, the hemogram shows leuko-

---

*) Koplik's spots may also be seen in ECHO virus infections. *The translators.*

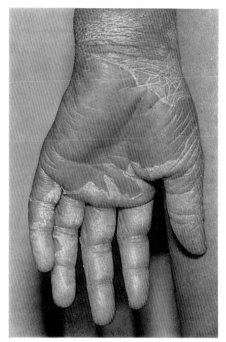

Fig. 1. Recurrent scarlatiniform erythema

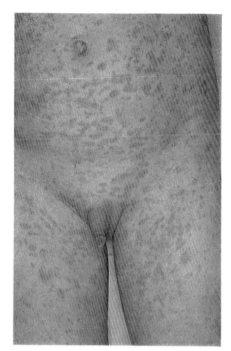

Fig. 3. Measles

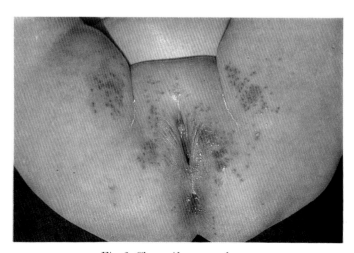

Fig. 2. Chancriform pyoderma

3

cytosis. Later there is a characteristic leukopenia with a shift to the left, and the absence of eosinophils is noted. The urine becomes diazopositive. Typical complications, such as otitis media, croup, bronchiolitis, pneumonia, and encephalitis, will not be discussed here. In regard to "*morbilli vesiculosi*" or the questionable existence of the so-called "*pemphigoid of measles,*" in our own experience (KÖTTGEN and KORTING) these represent instances of highly morbilloid-bullous Lyell's syndrome. This could be proved in one case, in which the patient later developed typical measles.

German measles (rubella)

This infectious disease, which is seen primarily in children from two to 10 years of age, is also caused by a virus. It can be responsible for fetal malformations (cataract, cardiac malformations, deafness, and so forth) if the mother becomes infected in the first trimester of pregnancy. Mild signs of an upper respiratory infection mark the onset of the disease. Swelling of the lymph nodes – chiefly the occipital-nuchal nodes – are a prominent sign. The hemogram shows a marked increase of plasma cells (5 to 10 per cent). The exanthem of rubella can best be compared to "rudimentary measles." The small macule of German measles, however, is slightly lighter and the individual lesion is smaller than that of measles. The exanthem may spread in crops but always extends in contiguity. It begins, just as measles, in the retroauricular region. The specificity of the exanthem was still denied by HEBRA and KAPOSI.

The exanthem of infectious mononucleosis may closely simulate that of rubella. The disease, however, begins with diphtheroid or Plaut-Vincent-like tonsillitis. The fever is higher. Other signs are generalized swelling of the lymph nodes, enlargement of the liver and spleen, definite lymphomonocytosis, and high leukocytosis. The diagnosis is corroborated by the heterophil antibody reaction (Paul-Bunnell test).

Scarlet fever (scarlatina)

Scarlet fever is caused by beta-hemolytic streptococci of group A (and perhaps an additional virus) and begins in the upper respiratory tract. Suddenly – this happens especially in cases of scarlet fever superimposed on wounds or burns – a flaming dusky redness of the pharynx develops, with dirty grayish tonsillar membranes. This is accompanied by high fever, rapid pulse, and vomiting. The exanthem, which soon follows, is observed initially on the inner aspects of the thighs, arms, and anterior axillary folds. Circumorally, the skin remains clear, in strong contrast to the flaming redness of the body. Additional findings are leukocytosis with a shift to the left, eosinophilia, Döhle's inclusion bodies, the presence of urobilinogen in the urine, blanching of the skin following injection of scarlet fever convalescent serum (Schultz-Charlton reaction), a positive Dick test, and a positive Rumpel-Leede test.

The so-called raspberry tongue reveals swollen papillae at the tip and the sides. The exanthem gives the impression of being a solid erythema, known to be a concomitant of high fever. On closer inspection, however, the exanthem is seen to consist of many closely

4

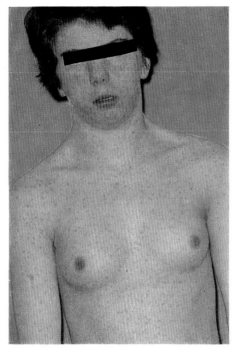

Fig. 4. Measles (characteristic facial appearance)

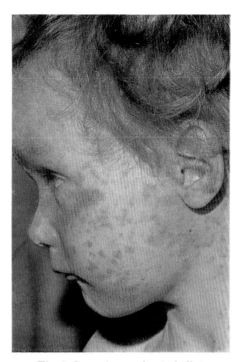

Fig. 6. German measles (rubella)

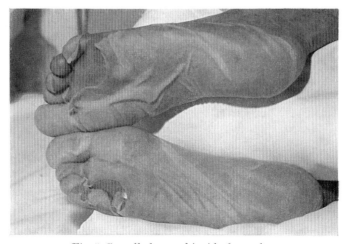

Fig. 5. So-called pemphigoid of measles

aggregated, small (to pinhead sized) light red or flaming red macules, which may temporarily become swollen. The skin between the lesions assumes a slightly yellowish hue. As early as one to two days later the eruption loses its characteristic appearance, and after one week has usually disappeared completely. Occasionally, however, the rash is followed, after two or three weeks, by characteristic branlike scales located on the hands, feet, and auricular pinnae; these scales peel off in large lamellae, or in a glovelike manner. There is no relationship between the intensity of the exanthem and this membranous desquamation. Other complications involving joints, heart, and kidneys will not be discussed here.

Erythema infectiosum (fifth disease)

Erythema infectiosum is seen in children under 14 years of age who initially present signs of an upper respiratory infection. The eruption begins on the cheeks with a mild erythema in butterfly distribution. This is followed by a discontinuous eruption, which spreads to distant areas and is arranged in reticular distribution or geographic maplike figures. The German name "ringlike rubella" refers to this arrangement. The eruption first appears on the extensor surface of the arms, later on the flexor aspect of the forearms, and finally over the buttocks. The palms and soles remain clear. The duration of the disease is about seven days.

Erythema infectiosum variabile

In August 1958 an exanthematous pandemic appeared in Kiel, Germany, and spread over wide areas of Germany (Rhein, Ruhr, Main, Neckar, Spree), Holland, and Switzerland. The disorder was erroneously named "blister disease." Later, an emulsifier of margarine was suspected of being the causative factor, and the disorder became known as "margarine disease." It was accompanied by subfebrile temperatures. The exanthem, frequently accompanied by violent itching, favored young girls and women. Children under 10 years of age remained conspicuously unaffected. The eruption had characteristics of both erythema infectiosum and erythema multiforme. The lesions were sometimes urticarial or hemorrhagic, and as in typhus and secondary syphilis, involved the palms. The disorder is no longer observed.

In connection with this explosive pandemic, which for a while was considered to be due to a virus, it should be noted that children in whom adenovirus and enterovirus could be isolated did have exanthems, among them roseola or morbilliform eruptions. But it could not be proved that the isolated viral agents were responsible for the exanthematous infections.

Erythema annulare rheumaticum

Today this exanthem is found only rarely among the cutaneous manifestations in rheumatics. It affects the upper abdomen almost exclusively, forming marginated and polycyclic erythematous rings. The exanthem is non-pruritic and subsides after a few days without

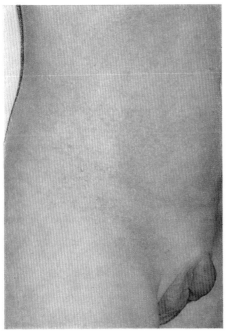

Fig. 7. Scarlet fever

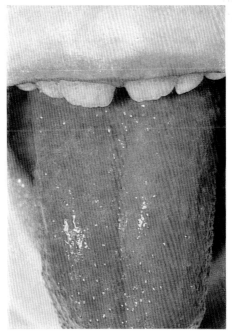

Fig. 8. The tongue in scarlet fever

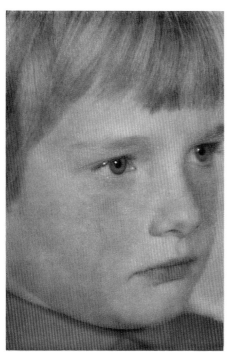

Fig. 9. Erythema infectiosum (butterfly
erythema of the face)

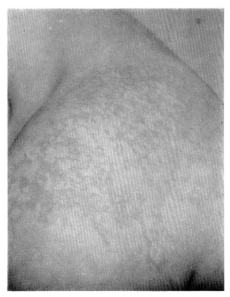

Fig. 10. Erythema infectiosum

sequelae. Longer duration is exceptional. The presence of this eruption indicates a florid cardiac complication of acute rheumatic fever. Recurrences have been observed. In any case, this exanthem, which formerly was supposed to be present in up to 60 per cent of patients suffering from carditis, represents "rheumatism's calling card, which, unfortunately, is presented too late" (FANCONI).

Erythema annulare centrifugum (Darier)

This erythema develops abruptly but then persists for months or years without much change. Spreading centrifugally and extremely slowly, it forms small and large polycyclic gyrate configurations. It is most probably related to other rare erythematous eruptions such as erythema gyratum perstans or erythema gyratum repens (GAMMEL). A certain variability exists: induration, scaling, blisters, and even purpura and telangiectases have occasionally been observed. The etiology of a single case often remains unsolved. Mild toxic effects are most probably responsible for this "id" or "dermatophytid" reaction. It is, however, imperative to rule out underlying visceral neoplasias, leukemias, and reticuloendothelioses.

Acrodermatitis papulosa eruptiva infantilis (Gianotti-Crosti syndrome)

This acrodermatosis was originally reported from Milan, Italy, in 1955 but has been observed in several European countries, including Germany. The eruption is accompanied by enlarged lymph nodes and a large liver (transaminases!). It is monotonously lichenoid and papular, and spreads on the extremities from the distal to the proximal parts. The trunk and the perioral, nasolabial and periocular areas are not affected. Occasionally, one sees a discrete purpuric note. Chiefly affected are boys between two and four years of age. The hemogram shows increased lymphomonocytes; immunoelectrophoretically, elevation of the ceruloplasmin (own observation) is observed. After a long duration the lesions disappear and do not recur.

Acrodermatitis enteropathica

This dermatosis, which probably has been often misdiagnosed as epidermolysis bullosa hereditaria, seems to occur throughout the world. Two hundred cases have been observed. Children in their first years of life are affected, and, quite frequently the disease appears in several children of one family. Neither sex is especially favored. The eruption is characterized by erythema with superimposed vesiculopustules or crusts. It occurs in a strikingly symmetric fashion, chiefly near all the body openings and the distal parts of the extremities; therefore, it was given the name acrodermatitis. Pustular paronychias, dystrophies of the nail, and alopecia are pathognomonic features. Blepharoconjunctivitis with photophobia is less frequently observed. Diarrhea, however, is almost always present. Characteristically, Candida albicans is a frequent secondary invader. Refractory to ordinary drugs and of grave prognosis, the disorder responds promptly to chinolin derivatives (SCHLOMOWITZ) such as

8

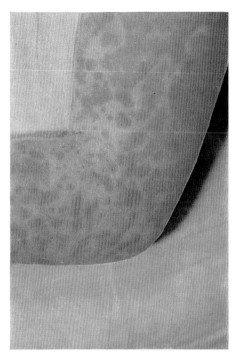

Fig. 11. Erythema infectiosum variabile (margarine disease)

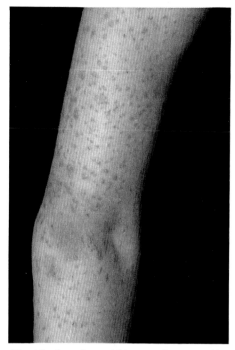

Fig. 12. Acrodermatitis papulosa eruptiva infantilis (Gianotti-Crosti syndrome)

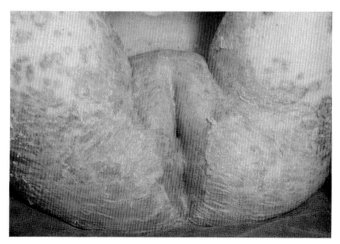

Fig. 13. Acrodermatitis enteropathica

Diodoquin (diiodohydroxyquinoline) and Entero-vioform (iodochlorhydroxyquin). The diagnosis can almost be made on the basis of the patient's response to this therapy. The cause of the disorder may be a genetically determined enzyme defect, which is also responsible for the simultaneous intestinal involvement.

Erythema chronicum migrans

The initial lesion is a single macule, which over a period of months slowly develops into an extended erythema (although there is a tendency to spontaneous regression). The resulting ringed lesions may develop polycyclic borders. While the trunk and extremities are sites of predilection, the face may also be affected. Middle-aged individuals are favored. The eruption is as a rule not pruritic but may occasionally be associated with headaches, subfebrile temperatures, or mild meningeal signs. In analogy to acrodermatitis chronica atrophicans and lymphocytoma, the eruption follows a bite by a tick, Ixodes ricinus, which is found on trees in wooded areas in Germany in May or September. The bite causes no pain. It is still not clear whether erythema migrans represents a viral infection or a reaction to the toxic saliva of the tick.

Erythema multiforme

The typical lesion is a round, light red spot with concentric zones and varying degrees of exudate creating the diagnostically characteristic iris or target lesion. Confluent lesions may form gyrate forms. The dorsa of the hands, extensor surfaces of the forearms, the face, the neck, and the mucous membrane of the lips are sites of predilection. If the oral or genital mucosa are more affected, involvement of the flexor rather than the extensor aspects of the extremities is the rule.

This classic form has many synonyms which stress special characteristics, such as the preferred location at body openings (ectodermosis erosiva pluriorificialis, FIESSINGER-RENDU, 1917, and dermatostomatitis, BAADER, 1925). If there is general involvement, particularly with pneumonia and nephritic complications, pediatricians favor the concept of the Stevens-Johnson syndrome.

The disorder either occurs in a "genuine" form, with atypic pneumonic complications and an increase in cold agglutinins, or else it represents a polyetiologic syndrome, which has been provoked by drug allergies or infections. The latter occurs more frequently. In the "herpetid" form of erythema multiforme, exquisitely small iris lesions are present. Occasionally, hematologic disorders such as leukemia begin as erythema multiforme. Uncomplicated cases, especially the recurrent type, however, have infrequently been provoked by "physical" agents such as x-rays and certain atmospheric weather conditions. Even HEBRA pointed to the autumn-spring peak (KEINING: typus annuus) of the disorder. In other cases the streptogenic cause of the disease is emphasized by an initial sore throat. Etiologically, we are dealing in most cases with a toxic or allergic-hyperergic reaction of the cutaneous vessels as far down as the arterioles.

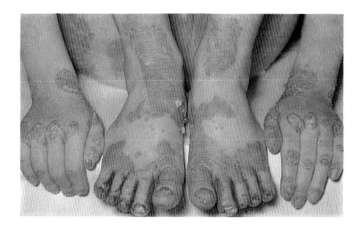

Fig. 14. Acrodermatitis
enteropathica

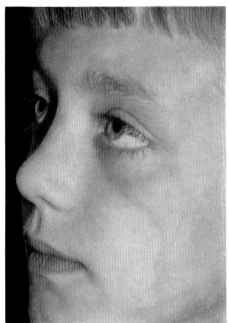

Fig. 15. Erythema migrans

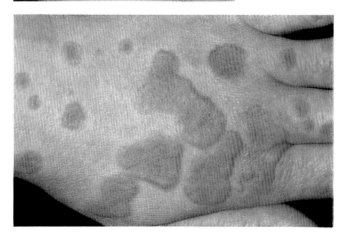

Fig. 16. Erythema multiforme

Erythema elevatum diutinum

In 1894 CROCKER and WILLIAMS described this rare disorder which resembles erythema multiforme as well as granuloma annulare. It also affects the extensor surface of the extremities, especially the hands and the skin over the joints. The lesions are rather monomorphic, developing subacutely or subchronically into round or polycyclic tuberous infiltrates of a blue-red hue, frequently with a central depression.

Formerly, the disease was classified into two subgroups: middle-aged women exhibited the Hutchinson type, which led to ulcerations with scarring; the Bury type affected women and children. The lesions did not last long, but tended to subside and recur, especially in summer. HERZBERG believes that extracellular cholesterosis (KERL-URBACH) represents a variation of erythema elevatum diutinum that is characterized by secondary lipid inclusion.

Erythema nodosum

Whereas erythema multiforme frequently affects the upper extremities, erythema nodosum, the tuberous erythema, favors the lower half of the body and its deeper cutaneous vessels, that is, the deep cutis and septa of the subcutaneous fatty layers. Successive infiltrates, which may be as large as walnuts, are characteristically either superficial (contusiform) or else subcutaneous, tender, and occasionally plaquelike. Under the name erythema nodosum migrans BÄFVERSTEDT described a special erysipelas-like eruption which may "migrate." In children, the extensor aspects of the arms, and even the face, may be the sites of the eruption. Fever is not uncommon. The etiologic relationship of erythema nodosum in childhood to tuberculosis will be discussed in a later chapter (see tuberculids). All four venereal diseases (syphilis, gonorrhea, lymphopathia venereum, and granuloma inguinale), as well as the dermatomycoses, sarcoidosis, rheumatic fever, Hodgkin's disease, and to a lesser degree reticuloendothelioses and leukemia may show erythema nodosum. Most frequently, however, it represents a "toxic exanthem."

Acrodynia (Feer's disease)

In 1914 SWIFT described this disorder as "Erythrödem"; CLUBBE named it "pink disease." Also known as WESTON's acrodynia and FEER's vegetative neurosis, it is characterized by acral cyanosis and large lamellar palmoplantar desquamations or macerations. Not infrequently, exanthems are present on the trunk and extremities. The rather impressive picture may be complicated by an ulcerative enanthem, hypertonia, tachycardia, muscle weakness, profuse sweating, and a depressive mood with crying spells. Moreover, since the disease has always seemed to be surpassed in importance by the clinical manifestations of ergotism and ustilaginism, and with the recognition of the disorder as a late neuro-allergic reaction to mercury (FANCONI, BOTSZTEJN, and SCHENKER: calomel disease), it has lost much of its significance.

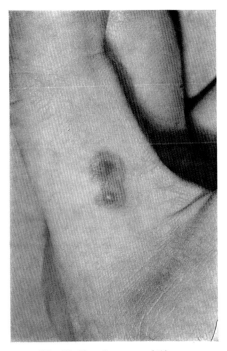

Fig. 17. Erythema multiforme

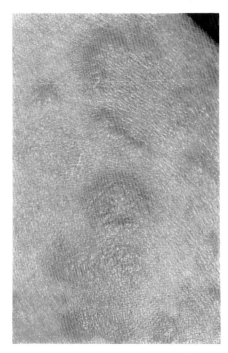

Fig. 18. Erythema elevatum diutinum

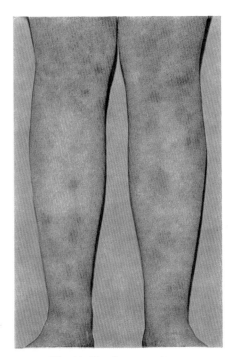

Fig. 19. Erythema nodosum

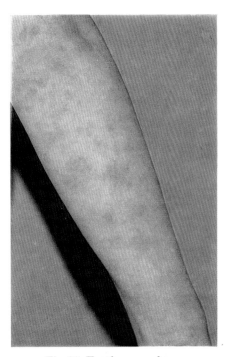

Fig. 20. Erythema nodosum

Toxic-allergic exanthems

Many diseases that are important in differential diagnosis in everyday practice may be grouped together under the heading "allergies." J. JADASSOHN expressed this in another way: "The toxicodermas and drug eruptions today occupy the place which 50 years ago was taken up by the great imitator, syphilis." These cutaneous reactions of intolerance do not often point conspicuously to the causative agent. For example, the eruption recurring every time at the same spot and therefore called a fixed drug eruption (mucosa of the lips, oral cavity, and glans penis), may be caused by legumen, pyrazolones, or phenolphthalein; acneiform eruptions may occur secondary to administration of halogens, cortisone, vitamin D, or anti-malarial compounds. The eruption following certain drugs (hydralazine, griseofulvin) masks lupus erythematosus. Certain other toxic-allergic exanthems require additional trigger factors such as exposure to light. The eruptive reaction to Istizin is a toxic erythema of the buttocks resulting from transformation of Istizin into Cignolin in the colon (IPPEN). Drug reactions to iodine or bromide often assume a vegetating aspect. Most of the drug eruptions, however, are of a stereotyped character, either scarlatiniform, or morbilliform. Therefore, when first observed, and without the benefit of a history, these reaction appear to be of unclear origin. In addition, the cutaneous intolerance is not infrequently associated with other general signs such as drug fever, arthralgias, a precipitous drop of leukocytes and blood platelets, and hemolysis. Drug reactions also tend to appear relatively late. An eruption caused by Salvarsan (arsphenamine) may appear on the ninth day. The cutaneous complications of penicillin may also appear late.

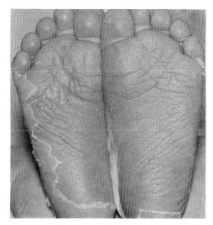
Fig. 21. Acrodynia (Feer's disease)

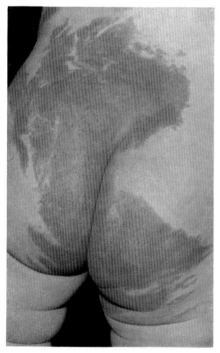
Fig. 22. Dermatitis following ingestion of
Istizin

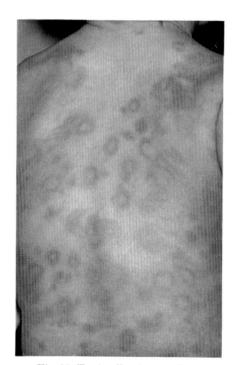
Fig. 23. Toxic-allergic exanthem

2. Erythematosquamous Dermatoses

Psoriasis vulgaris

"Parakeratotic diathesis" (ŠAMBERGER) or "essential parakeratosis" (GRÜNEBERG) is due to an exaggerated increase of epidermopoiesis (LORINCZ). This is evident not only from the distinct increase in the oxidizing processes (GANS, BUHMANN) or the sulfhydryl groups (ZINGSHEIM), but chiefly from an alteration in DNA synthesis and the resulting disturbance in the keratinization process. A biologic underformation (KYRLE) of keratinization, that is, parakeratosis, results. According to this concept, psoriasis is primarily an epidermal process. Psoriasis also represents, however, an *erythemato*squamous dermatosis, since after the characteristic lamellar scales are removed, a saturated erythema of long duration with a dewlike "drop" of blood (sign of AUSPITZ) becomes evident. Abnormally long capillaries or even glomerulo-like capillary convolutions are responsible for this phenomenon. In spite of the characteristic single lesion, the appearance of the eruption can vary greatly, as is evident from its various descriptions: psoriasis vulgaris, punctata, guttata, nummularis, discoides, annularis, geographica, gyrata, and so forth.

Psoriatic erythroderma without typical individual lesions represents the maximal ecto-dermal variation, whereas *psoriasis arthropathica*, which presumably is genetically con-trolled, represents the maximal mesenchymatous variation. Psoriasis arthropathica slightly favors the male sex and is present in about 1.5 per cent of all psoriatics. While characteristic rheumatoid serologic factors are absent, a reduction of IgM globulins is occasionally observed on electrophoresis. Caution should be taken in treating these arthropathies with chloroquine derivatives, since under such treatment the psoriatic process may exacerbate. Regression of the single lesion may result in either hyperpigmentation or depigmentation, the so-called leukoderma psoriaticum, to be distinguished from leukoderma psoriaticum spurium, which follows administration of certain medicaments. White perifocal zones point to imminent healing (*ring of* WORONOFF); red halos, on the other hand, signify progression. Favored sites are the extensor surfaces of the extremities. Occasionally, however, an inverse type which favors the flexor surfaces is seen. Frequently, the scalp and the face are involved (for example, in the presence of light and heat factors), with emphasis on the frontal hairline. The nails (in 15 per cent of patients with psoriasis vulgaris and in 80 to 90 per cent of patients with psoriasis arthropathica) show pitting, have subungual debris, and are parakeratotically

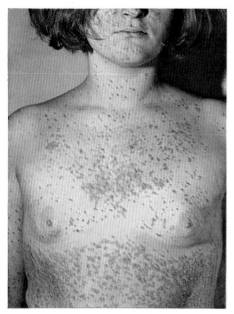

Fig. 24. Guttate psoriasis vulgaris

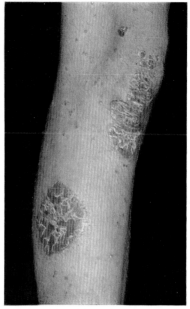

Fig. 25. Discoid psoriasis vulgaris

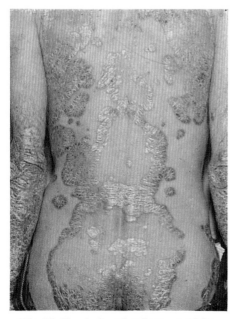

Fig. 26. Psoriasis vulgaris geographica

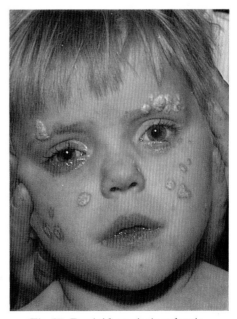

Fig. 27. Rupioid psoriasis vulgaris

17

discolored or crumbled. Not infrequently, the nail is secondarily invaded mycotically, as is also observed in intertriginous psoriasis (diaper psoriasis), which tends toward monilial superinfection. In psoriasis vulgaris, there is itching with the elevated plaster-like lesions and even more with the yellowish-white lesions in the presence of hyperuricemia.

One must distinguish between pustular psoriasis and the acral form restricted to the palmo-plantar surfaces. In differential diagnosis, ANDREWS's bacterid, which may represent transformed palmoplantar psoriasis, and parakeratosis pustulosa must be considered. Pustular psoriasis over the distal finger joints seems to be identical with acrodermatitis continua suppurativa (HALLOPEAU), while psoriasis pustulosa in pregnancy is called "impetigo herpetiformis."

Psoriasis vulgaris may for years remain stationary. Such chronic lesions are located chiefly over the sacral region. Psoriasis vulgaris is characterized by KÖBNER's or KREIBICH's phenomenon, an isomorphic scratch effect, and a certain "isopathic" tendency to healing (SCHMIDT-LABAUME). Showing irregular dominance, it may be multifactorial with a thres-hold effect. Psoriatic manifestations may depend distinctly on environmental factors, such as strong light, or on endogenous changes such as endocrine turning points (menarche), febrile infections, or certain metabolic abnormalities (obesity, diabetes mellitus*). In any case, the initial changes of psoriasis may occur in childhood or even infancy. Statistics put psoriasis in childhood at 10 per cent of all cases of psoriasis. The most frequent age for the onset of psoriasis, however, is between the ages of 20 and 40.

The Parapsoriasis Group

In 1902 BROCQ classified three dermatoses as "parapsoriases." As ARNDT remarked, however, these dermatoses hardly resemble psoriasis and are pathogenetically not related to it.

Pityriasis lichenoides chronica (Parapsoriasis guttata)

This distinctly chronic dermatosis of long duration presents with almost stationary, typical reddish-brown papules which are initially copper colored. The papules can easily be distinguished from those of lichen planus, but may resemble the papules of secondary syphilis. The mature papules are covered by wafer- or collodion-like scales, which can be lifted intact. After removal of the scale, which is thicker in the center than at the periphery, red, saturated, noninfiltrated areas remain.

Also typical of this dermatosis are chronicity, resistance to therapy, absence of symptoms, and, occasionally, healing with leukoderma. In adolescents this classic form is seen inter-

---

* In psoriatic patients diabetes mellitus does not occur more often than in controls. The trans-lators.

18

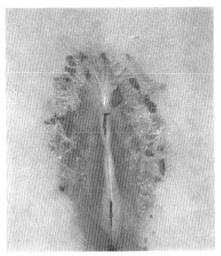

Fig. 28. Intertriginous psoriasis

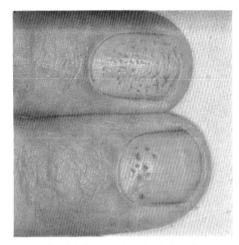

Fig. 31. Psoriatic stippled nails

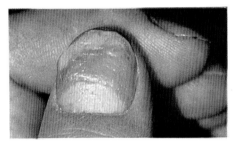

Fig. 32. Psoriatic yellowish (oily)
discoloration of the nail plate

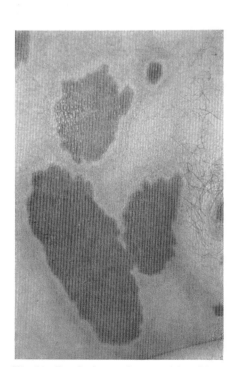

Fig. 29. Psoriatic erythema with white
halo (ring of Woronoff)

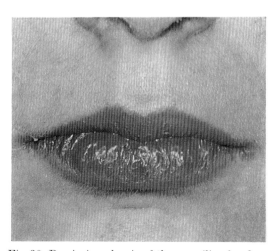

Fig. 30. Psoriasis vulgaris of the vermilion border

spersed with varicelliform, pustular, vesiculohemorrhagic, or necrotic elements. TOUTON described seborrheic types and GOTTRON acute-vesicular types. The lichenoid and varioliform or varicelliform variety, not infrequently observed, was reported by MUCHA in 1916 and HABERMANN in 1925. Lately, this type has been considered to represent an allergic vasculitis, since such changes as endothelial swelling, necrosis of the wall of the vessel, obliterations, and so forth are observed. This acute type apparently occurs in connection with upper respiratory infections and regresses much faster than the chronic type.

Brocq's disease (Parapsoriasis en plaques)

In 1897 BROCQ described this dermatosis, naming it "érythrodermie pityriasique en plaques disséminées." The dermatosis is characterized by monotonous, yellowish-red, noninfiltrating, and occasionally slightly atrophic lesions covered with a fine scale. The lesions occur predominantly on the trunk and less frequently on the extremities, for the most part, in long stripes and only infrequently in round or oval arrangements. The lesions are not so discrete as those of seborrheic dermatitis; they may show a few nodules, such as those of lichen simplex, and after intense scratching punctate hemorrhagic lesions may become visible. Increasing swelling or infiltration of single lesions and pruritus suggest transformation into mycosis fungoides or premycosis.

Parakeratosis variegata (Parapsoriasis lichenoides)

In England R. CROCKER named this dermatosis lichen variegatus. It may begin as pityriasis lichenoides chronica, later developing into an elevated retiform pattern composed of confluent, hemispherical or polygonal, shiny, and often slightly scaling papules resembling lichen planus. After a long duration the lesions heal with slight atrophy. Individual cases have so little in common that it is doubtful whether we are dealing with an entity here.

Pityriasis rubra pilaris (Devergie)

This dermatosis was described in 1851 by DEVERGIE and was later identified with lichen ruber acuminatus by HEBRA. It affects not only children and adolescents but also persons around the fifth decade. Characteristic are closely aggregated, acuminate papules located at the hair follicles (especially over the dorsa of the fingers). Psoriasiform lesions develop over the elbows and erythematosquamous changes appear on the face, resulting in a fine, plaster of Paris-like cover over intense reddishness. Finally, there are frequently diffuse palmoplantar hyperkeratoses. Partial or generalized monotonously erythrodermic stages have been observed. Familial cases have been reported.

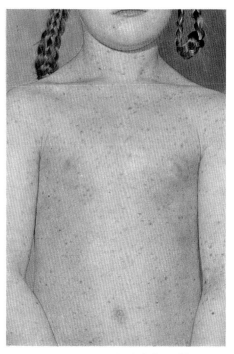

Fig. 33. Parapsoriasis lichenoides
chronica atrophicans

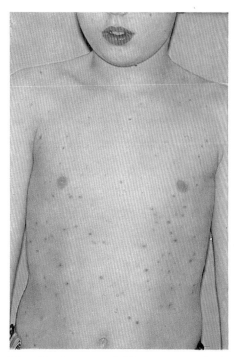

Fig. 34. Acute varioliform parapsoriasis

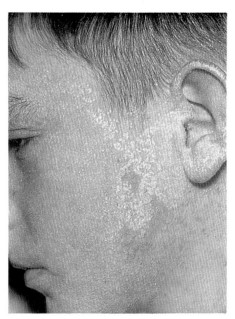

Fig. 35. Pityriasis rubra pilaris

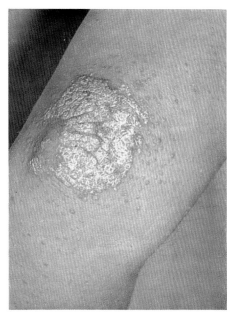

Fig. 36. Pityriasis rubra pilaris

21

Pityriasis rosea (Gibert, 1860)

Not infrequently, the manifestations of this disorder occur on the trunk in the projection toward the axillary fold. The multiple discrete lesions usually appear after a larger "herald patch." Located in the lines of cleavage, the lesions show slight scaling with a "collarette" at the margin. The face is usually spared. The lesions heal spontaneously but may leave a leukoderma. Children are often affected, but rarely before the second year of life. In some geographic areas, in Germany, for instance, there seems to be a peak in late fall, which may reach epidemic proportions. The disorder does not affect the general well-being of the patient but is often preceded by an upper respiratory infection, which suggests the possibility of a viral infection or a streptogenic id-reaction.

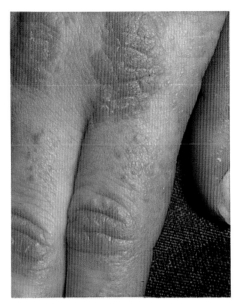

Fig. 37. Pityriasis rubra pilaris

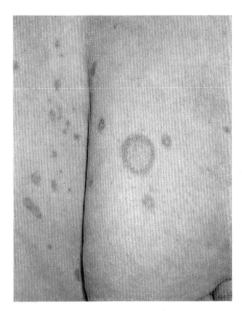

Fig. 38. Pityriasis rosea with typical
herald patch (primary plaque)

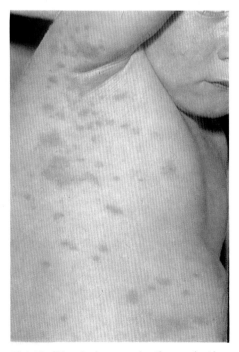

Fig. 39. Pityriasis rosea in the projection
toward the axilla

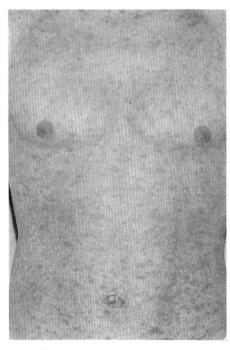

Fig. 40. Irritated pityriasis rosea

3. Eczema Group. Dermatitis

According to GOTTRON, eczema can be classified as common, seborrheic (bacterial), and endogenous. Common eczema (dermatitis venenata) is primarily the result of external conditions, whereas the seborrheic and endogenous eczemas are based on constitutional factors and affect different age groups (KORTING). Dermatitis venenata or contact dermatitis is characterized by erythematous patches which occur within a definite period of time, as a local response to external irritants. Vesicles may develop, followed by vesiculo-pustules. Later stages are characterized by scaling, crusts, and infiltration.

For the detection of the causative factor of common eczema, the skin should be exposed to test substances as outlined by J. JADASSOHN (1905) and BRUNO BLOCH (1911). The reaction of the skin to the test substances presents histologically an "eccème en miniature." The test is performed by applying a three-layered plaster with the test substance to normal skin (otherwise there will be false positive results). Histologically, the cells responsible for the eczematous infiltration are not only lymphocytes, but also monocytes (BANDMANN); toxic reactions of the skin, on the other hand, show primarily polymorphonuclear leukocytes (NEXMAND). It is important to use only safe concentrations when performing the skin tests. When there is doubt, a sufficient number of individuals with normal skin should be tested as controls.

The initial lesions of *seborrheic eczema* (UNNA, 1887) are yellowish-brown erythematous patches with peripheral exudation. These patches may be symmetrically or asymmetrically

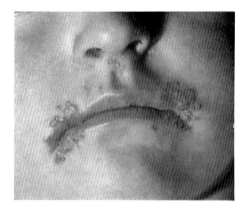

Fig. 41. Perioral dermatitis (after eating a green apple)

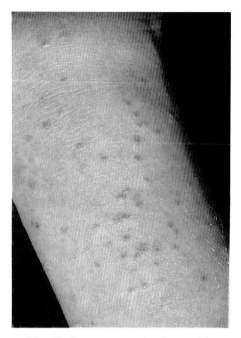

Fig. 42. Common papular dermatitis

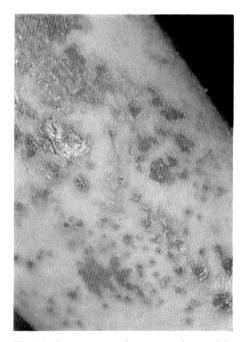

Fig. 43. Common erythematous dermatitis

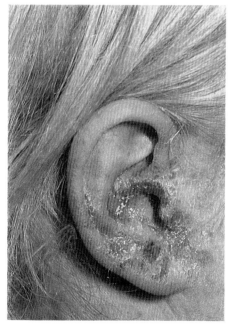

Fig. 44. Impetiginized dermatitis of the ear

arranged. They show a preference for intertriginous areas, which are richly supplied with sweat and oil glands. A pyogenic focus of infection may act as a trigger. In addition seborrheic eczema shows more of a tendency to develop small patches which become widespread by continuous extension (microbid) than the other two types of eczema. At first, round or oval, petaloid, polycyclic, punctate, perifollicular lesions may arise, simultaneously or in succession; their edges are sharply demarcated ("pityriasis marginata"). The faces of children exhibit a minimal discoid dermatitis, which often presents only as a pseudovitiligo; this is the so-called "minimal variant" of preseborrhea, seen chiefly if hypertrophic pharyngeal adenoids are present and if provoked by spring sunlight. This condition is also called leaping dermatitis ("dartre volante"), pityriasis simplex (WILLAN), or streptodermia superficialis (JADASSOHN).

The patient with the endogenous atopic type of eczema may suffer at the same time from asthma or vasomotoric rhinitis, or may show one of these conditions at another time. Usually, there is a family history of one or all of these conditions.

Synonyms for endogenous eczema (a term coined by GOTTRON, KORTING) are asthma-eczema, prurigo-eczema (SABOURAUD), prurigo Besnier, early and late exudative eczematoid (ROST), neurodermatitis disseminata, lately called neurodermatitis constitutionalis (BORELLI and SCHNYDER), and finally "atopic dermatitis" (PERRY, COCA). The very first exudative phase with spongiosis of the endogenous eczema is the infantile facial eczema. There are many somewhat confusing terms for this condition: crusta lactea, croûte laiteuse, tâches de lait, cradle cap, and so forth.

Infantile eczema characteristically affects the lateral aspects of the face (this is the initial lesion of 70 per cent of all cases of endogenous eczema). During nursery and school days the *flexural eczema* is seen in 80 per cent on the antecubital and 40 per cent on the popliteal folds. Still later we speak of the disseminated eczematous lichen simplex-like eruption. Chronic papular urticaria or the prurigo reaction represents the last stage. During the third decade of life this occasionally monomorphic prurigo phase resembles the papular urticaria variety. In the fourth decade one encounters the large nodes of prurigo nodularis; this condition is occasionally complicated by lymphadenitis causing large "prurigo buboes."

Formerly (before the corticosteroids), the lichenified areas of endogenous eczema were characterized by circumscribed, striated rectangular patches; polycyclic borders, when present, pointed to interaction with a secondary bacterial infection. After prolonged local or systemic corticosteroid therapy, the originally sharp border of the lichenified lesions becomes less distinct. However, even after many weeks of treatment with corticosteroid ointment, a distinct brownish-yellow, or peculiarly dull, reddish-gray lichenification remains. Sometimes the color is that of seborrhea, but the periphery fails to give the exudative appearance of the eczematized seborrheic eczema.

The different phases of atopic eczema (cradle cap, extensive lichenification, lichen simplex chronicus nodules, and papular lesions of prurigo) point to the absence of characteristic histologic features.

Beyond the fortieth year of life only about 3 per cent of patients with previous atopic eczema still show cutaneous manifestations. Ichthyotic skin may be an exception. Examinations 20 years later of patients who have had atopic eczema since childhood show cutaneous changes in only about one-quarter, and asthmatic or spastic-bronchitic signs in about half the patients. The dry skin of patients with atopic eczema should not be considered to be synonymous with genuine ichthyosis vulgaris. The latter shows platelike scales joined in linear or rhomboid figures in typical locations, other areas of the body not being involved.

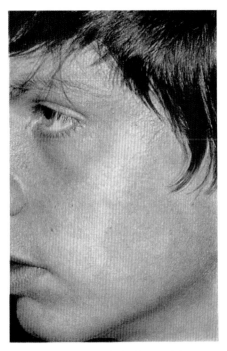

Fig. 45. Seborrheic dermatitis
(Pityriasis alba)

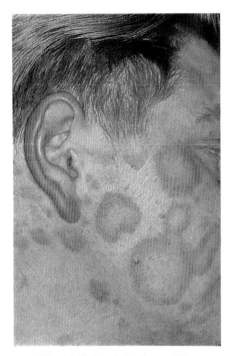

Fig. 46. Seborrheic dermatitis
(Pityriasis marginata)

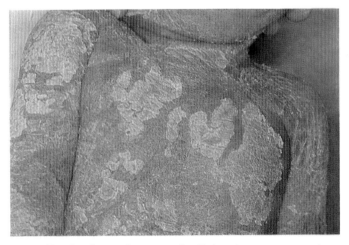

Fig. 47. Erythroderma desquamativa Leiner (most severe variant
of seborrheic dermatitis in childhood)

27

Furthermore, the patient with atopic eczema possesses characteristic features or stigmata, such as a fur cap-like hairline, a sallow colored skin, white dermographia, delayed erythematous response, broken-off hairs of the lateral portion of the eyebrows (Hertoghe's sign), oligobradyhidrosis, increased reactivity of the arrectores pilorum, and delayed neutralization of alkali. Rare ocular signs are dermatogenous cataract, keratoconus, and detachment of the retina. Another peculiarity is improvement of the skin disorder in mild summers, and aggravation in winter. There is frequently a definite dependence on climate; high mountains or territory close to the ocean are favorable. Acute, prognostically grave complications occur if the individual with endogenous eczema is exposed to smallpox vaccine or herpes simplex virus (eczema vaccinatum or eczema herpeticum). The fatality rate in uncomplicated endogenous eczema is low, but death in children with infantile eczema may result from myocarditis, encephalitis, enterocolitis, and later in life from status asthmaticus.

All three types of eczema (common, seborrheic, endogenous) may appear as early as in childhood. It is therefore erroneous to consider the separate classification of infantile eczema (childhood eczema, Moro, 1932; eczema infantum verum, Finkelstein, 1935). Certain forms of eczema, however, are peculiar to childhood, such as the erythrodermia desquamativa (Carl Leiner, 1908). This condition is the most severe variant of seborrheic dermatitis in childhood.

Leiner's erythroderma starts between the first and second months of life, apparently without pruritus or blister formation. Spreading quickly to the buttocks and scalp, it clears up without interruption within a few weeks. It is characterized by large, scaly, vivid red or yellow-red, erythematous areas. As a rule, there is no swelling of the lymph nodes, but there are almost always intestinal disturbances with thin mucous stools, tachycardia, an enlarged liver, and hypoproteinemia.

In differential diagnosis one has to consider atopic erythroderma, which is characterized by a shiny red appearance of the skin and little infiltration. Lymphadenopathy soon becomes a prominent sign. The white dermographia typical of the atopic eczema of later life cannot be elicited. Differential diagnosis between an atopic eczema and eczematous reactions seen in *ectodermal dysplasia (anhidrosis hypotrichotica)* and in *phenylketonuria (oligophrenia phenylpyruvica* Fölling) is difficult; the diagnosis of the latter condition is aided by the presence of a light complexion, follicular keratoses, and frequently observed photosensitivity. The combination of atopic diathesis with congenital ichthyosiform erythrodermia and trichorrhexis invaginata is known as Netherton's disease. The Wiskott-Aldrich syndrome, on the other hand, denotes chronic eczematoid cutaneous changes, initially more seborrheic-like, which are in later life more lichenified. Other signs are hemorrhages (petechiae, suffusions, hemorrhea) and thrombocytopenia, with an otherwise normal hemogram.

The treatment of children who have eczema, particularly the endogenous types, with special diets (smoked bacon, milk mixtures, and so forth) has been disappointing. Nevertheless, if cow's milk causes an exacerbation it can be substituted by goat's milk, condensed milk, or soybean protein. (There are instances of intolerance to the latter, as well.) In rare cases in early infancy, elimination of egg white may be necessary, but much more important is the avoidance of contact with wool. Otherwise the treatment of the aforementioned types of eczema depends on the respective stages of development and the condition of the skin, which may require either fat-poor or fatty ointment bases. The modern local treatment of eczema with corticosteroid ointments does not always result in complete regression, so that conventional therapy with ichthyol, tumenol, coal tar, and so forth has not become completely obsolete. (X-ray therapy has been abandoned.) When commercial cortisone ointments are applied at a distance from mucous membranes and only on limited areas, they may be used on children for some time without danger of significant side effects.

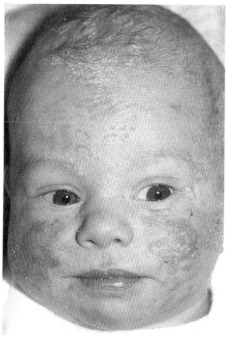

Fig. 48. Neurodermitis disseminata, atopic
dermatitis; cradle cap

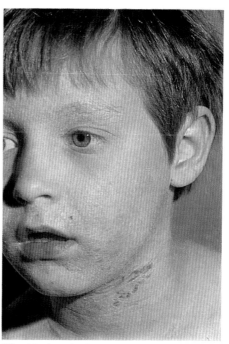

Fig. 49. Atopic dermatitis. Thinning of the
lateral part of the eyebrows (Hertoghe's
sign)

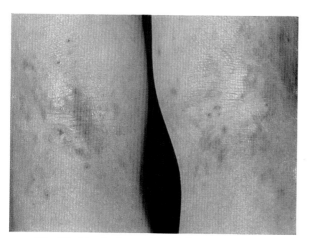

Fig. 50. Atopic dermatitis. "Flexural eczema"

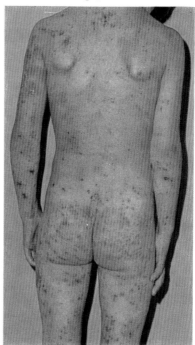

Fig. 51. Atopic dermatitis.
Disseminated eczematous lichenoid manifestations

29

Lichen simplex chronicus (Neurodermatitis circumscripta)

Lichen simplex chronicus (VIDAL, 1886) is not a manifestation of endogenous eczema, but up to the present time it has again and again been misdiagnosed as an abortive or atypical type of endogenous eczema. The fact that the patient with endogenous eczema may show primary lichenification and lesions somewhat similar to those of lichen simplex chronicus, does not permit the conclusion that the two conditions belong together. Lichen simplex or neurodermatitis circumscripta is not a familial disease. It occurs in isolated areas, usually for the first time in later life. Lichen simplex is dependent primarily on functional disorders of the gastrointestinal tract (anacidity, and so forth) and not on climate or season. Moreover, its location points to trauma (friction). In other words, lichen simplex fails to show a recognizable genetic basis, a development from childhood eczema, or a more than accidental combination with asthma and cataracts. Lichen simplex presents round, plane, pinhead sized – rarely somewhat larger (obtuse) – papules, which expand centrally to form patches of primary lichenification, in the periphery exhibiting a washed-out, dirty brown pigmentation. This completes the triple morphology. Among adolescent girls lichen simplex chronicus, as described here, occurs in the vulval region, in which it presents hyperkeratotic verrucous changes. Causative factors which may play a role here are intense traumatic rubbing, vaginal discharge, dribbling of urine, infestation with parasites, diabetes mellitus, and other factors.

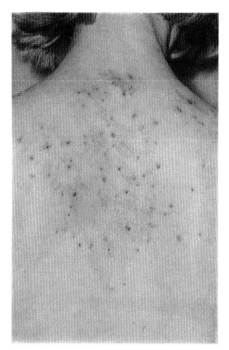

Fig. 52. Atopic dermatitis. Prurigo
type ("Prurigo leukodystrophica")

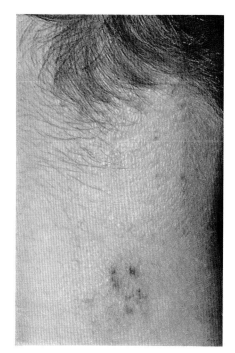

Fig. 53. Lichen simplex chronicus
(Neurodermatitis circumscripta)

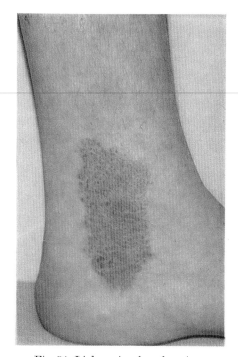

Fig. 54. Lichen simplex chronicus

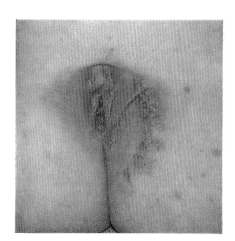

Fig. 55. Lichen simplex chronicus

31

4. Urticaria, Strophulus, and Prurigo

A *wheal* or *urticaria* shows an acute accumulation of initially pure fluid in the cutis. If the exudate becomes more cellular we speak of the papulovesicular manifestations of strophulus or lichen urticatus. The papule of prurigo shows the urticarial lesion to have finally become exquisitely cellular and interspersed with eosinophils. Because of this progressive development, these dermatoses – urticaria, strophulus, and prurigo – are discussed together.

Urticaria

Urticaria can appear at all ages, including infancy. In most cases pruritus is a prominent symptom. Because of varying osmotic pressure the eruption varies from fleeting red to porcelain-white annular or gyrate wheals. Penicillin given 8 to 10 days previously is the main culprit in urticaria of long duration with repeatedly new evanescent wheals. An acute onset is usually a sign of a drug or food allergy. Fruit (apples or apricots) is often responsible. In children and adolescents, products of disintegrated protein and inhalants play a smaller role than intestinal parasites (ascaris or trichuris). We are dealing with angioneurotic or Quincke's edema if the larynx and large symmetric areas of the face and neck become involved. Occasionally, this eruption is accompanied by intermittent swelling of the joints. In giant urticaria, or Quincke's edema, the larynx and glottis are the sites of edema and there is a danger of suffocation. Not infrequently, this complication is seen in several members of a family. It is possible that the individuals lack an inhibitor of esterase of the first component of the complement.

Physical urticaria (DUKE, 1924) can be caused by pressure, light, heat, cold, perspiration, and effort, among other factors. One individual may show several forms of physical urticaria (for example, urticaria from heat and from fatigue). *Cold urticaria* can become dangerous if diving into cold water in summertime causes anaphylactic shock. (Whether cold urticaria may be due to gastrointestinal foci of infection is questionable. The translators.) One has to keep in mind that edematous states similar to those in the skin can occur in inner organs, resulting in an increase of cerebral pressure or in disturbances of cardiac conduction. Clinically, physical urticaria is characterized by relatively small lesions.

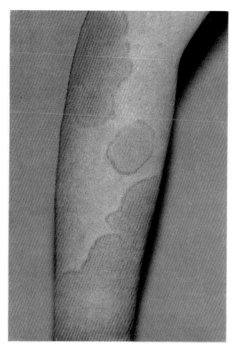

Fig. 56. Urticaria

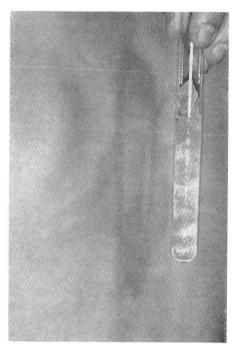

Fig. 57. Cold urticaria

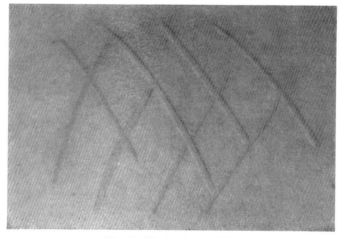

Fig. 58. Urticaria factitia

33

Pressure urticaria apparently requires an additional trigger of heat rather than cold. It must be differentiated from *urticaria factitia*, the red dermographia which is provoked by pronounced stroking of the upper part of the body; white dermographia occurs predominantly on the caudal part of the body, especially in the patient with endogenous eczema. Red dermographia is, by the way, not an expression of "allergy" but a stigma of a special nervous, vagotonic disposition.

Strophulus

In children, the papulovesicular lesion of strophulus persists for days, favoring the palms, soles, and buttocks. Histologically, it represents a seropapule. After the first three months of life infants may show light red eruptions of scant small nodules at the time of dentition. In such instances the face, which is usually spared, may become involved. Attacks of strophulus which are characterized by exacerbations of itching at night are generally caused by insect bites, the central bleeding mark being due to the bite. The improvement of children with strophulus in a hospital (SIEMENS: sanatio spontanea nosocomialis) also points to this parasitic origin. Infestation with animal parasites may also act as a trigger. In any case, a susceptibility to particular foods does not play a role.

Prurigo

In a few persons the prurigo papule represents a distinct individual reaction in response to various etiologic factors.

Being a lentil-sized, skin-colored, deep lying nodule, it is better felt than seen. It causes severe itching, and is for this reason frequently excoriated and covered with a small hemorrhagic crust. Healing with scarring is the rule. In older people, the prurigo papule is regularly associated with keratosis pilaris and ichthyosiform skin; characteristic of the eruption in a child is a tendency to develop enlarged lymph nodes, "prurigo ferox." Prurigo in adolescents has not infrequently begun in early childhood. Prurigo involves the extensor surfaces of the extremities. As in strophulus the face is spared. If different cutaneous changes are present simultaneously, we are dealing with "prurigo multiformis." In cases of endogenous eczema, the prurigo stage usually constitutes the last cutaneous reaction, the final stage. Prurigo lesions in dermatitis herpetiformis (DUHRING) are of short duration. In prurigo, more frequently than in other "skin reactions," the adult patient exhibits a series of underlying causes, such as infestation with parasites, too little gastric juice, liver disorders, leukemia, or systemic reticuloendothelioses. Prurigo that consists of large nodules, particularly prurigo nodularis (HYDE), is rarely seen in childhood.

Urticaria papulosa chronica is observed at menopause more often than at menarche.

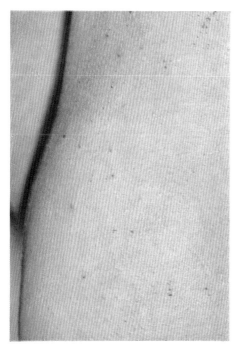

Fig. 59. Urticaria papulosa chronica

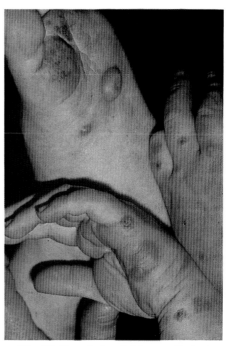

Fig. 60. Strophulus (Lichen urticatus)

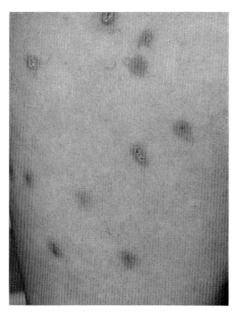

Fig. 61. Prurigo

5. Papular eruptions

Lichen planus

"Lichen" signifies a group of small nodules in a circumscribed area, having no tendency to further changes. The synonyms *lichen planus* (ERASMUS WILSON, 1859), *lichen ruber* (F. VON HEBRA, 1860), and *lichen ruber planus* (KAPOSI, 1877) describe a special cutaneous reaction consisting of plane, polygonal, and sharply circumscribed papules of a few millimeters with central dimples and a tendency to form plaques. The papules are firm, plane, and yellowish-pink to slate-colored. The dermatosis is rare in children. The surface of the lichen planus papule has epidermal and dermal components, and particularly in close grouping exhibits a milky-bluish, fern or spider web network (Wickham's striae). This clinical picture points to the histologic picture of the keratohyaline accentuation (Darier's granulosis), which is characteristic of lichen planus. A similar picture is seen on the mucous membranes. Some lesions of this severely pruritic nodular eruption are arranged in linear or striate fashion, representing an isomorphic response to scratching (Köbner's phenomenon). The favorite locations of the nodules are the wrists and forearms, the flanks, the sacral area, the genitals, and the extensor surfaces of the legs. On the legs the lesions occasionally become obtuse, hypertrophic, and verrucous. There are several varieties of this rather monomorphic eruption, such as an annular arrangement or transformation into a rather stubborn erythroderma or bullous eruption (lichen ruber pemphigoid). On the scalp, groups of follicular nodules are occasionally followed by pseudopeladic atrophic alopecias (Lassueur-Graham-Little syndrome).

The etiology and pathogenesis of lichen planus are unknown. Here again, the itching red papules constitute a specific skin reaction (BROCQ), illustrating that certain dermatoses are characterized not so much by certain causes but by specific skin responses. This means that the same dermatosis can evidently be provoked and formed by completely different causes. The cause of the individual instance of lichen planus, however, is still unsolved. In considering the pathogenesis of lichen planus, antitoxic rather than infectious factors have to be considered. A few familial cases have been seen. It is also known that environmental factors or drugs can cause a symptomatic outbreak of lichen planus. Formerly, the dermatosis was seen following treatment with gold or arsenic. During World War II "lichen tropicus" was noted following malaria suppressive therapy with atabrine. Recently, lichen planus was observed following exposure to color film developers.

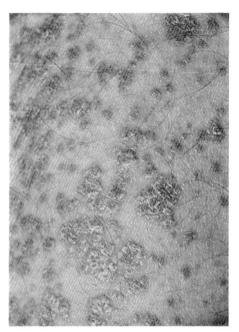

Fig. 62. Lichen planus

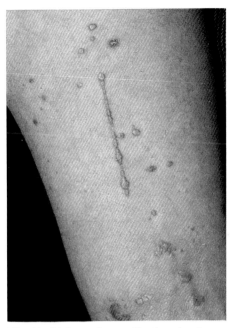

Fig. 63. Lichen planus (Koebner's phenomenon)

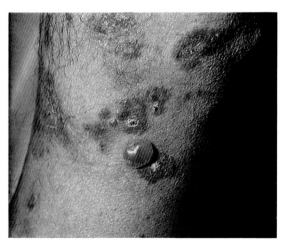

Fig. 64. Bullous lichen planus (Lichen planus pemphigoid)

Lichen nitidus

In contrast to lichen planus, which is rare in children, lichen nitidus, described in 1907 by F. PINKUS, represents a dermatosis affecting young people and infants almost exclusively. As PINKUS pointed out, we are dealing here with an eruption which rarely occurs in families, is of no practical significance, and most probably represents in spite of modified tuberculoid histologic changes ("granuloma nitidum") a variation of lichen ruber.

The initial lesion is a pinpoint to pinhead-sized, firm, smooth, round, polygonal, yellow-brown papule with a predilection for the shaft and glans of the penis, less frequently for the face or palms. The absence of itching, Wickham's striae, Köbner's phenomenon, and the variability of the lichen planus papule not only distinguish lichen nitidus from lichen planus but keep the lesions of lichen nitidus monomorphic.

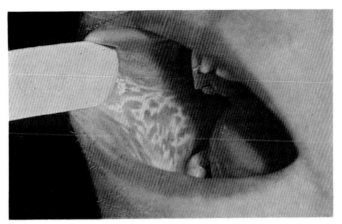

Fig. 65. Lichen planus of the oral mucosa

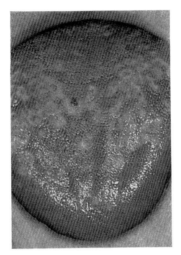

Fig. 66. Lichen planus of the
tongue

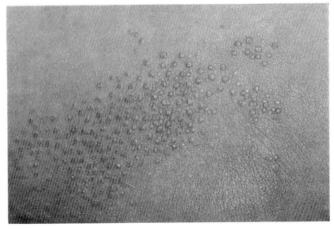

Fig. 67. Lichen nitidus

6. Acute Infectious Diseases of the Skin

Pyodermas

Cutaneous lesions caused by the hematogenic spread of common pyogenic organisms are relatively rare. Pyodermas (primary or secondary in pruriginous dermatoses), however, representing skin infections caused *externally* by streptococcus pyogenes or staphylococcus aureus, constitute 25 per cent of all skin diseases in children. Such manifestations occur in various layers of the skin (from epidermal and epidermocutaneous to deep cutaneous and subcutaneous layers) and are furthermore arranged either in wide areas without relation to the hair follicle or in special relation to the hair follicle. In infancy and childhood the duct of the eccrine sweat gland is a common site of infection. In adults, on the other hand, the hair follicles and the apocrine sweat glands are preferred sites. Other peculiarities of earliest childhood are the absence of the typical picture of impetigo contagiosa streptogenes in the infant, and absence of the tendency to blistering manifested by staphylococcus infections. Accordingly, the infant will show "pemphigus neonatorum" instead of a furuncle. Globonodular infiltrates, often misdiagnosed as furuncles, are really abscesses of the eccrine sweat glands (periporitis). The increased exudative reactivity of infants and small children is evident in the formation of bullae in response to various toxic and infectious agents, as in the reactions seen in syphilis and scabies or reactions to halogens.

This bullous type of reaction is not often observed in infants and small children. Certain classic bullous dermatoses, such as pemphigus vulgaris and dermatitis herpetiformis Duhring, do not occur in the newborn and hardly ever in early childhood.

40

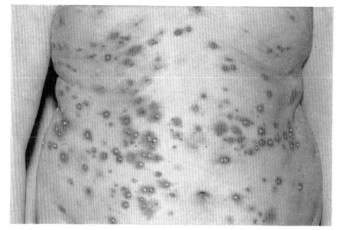

Fig. 68. Follicular impetigo (Wilson-Bockhart)

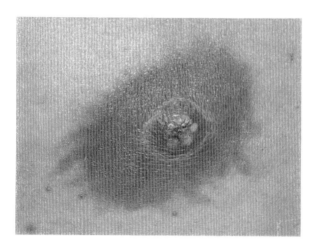

Fig. 69. Furuncle

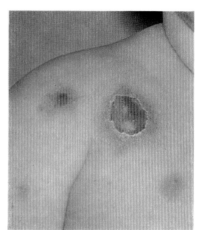

Fig. 70. Periporitis

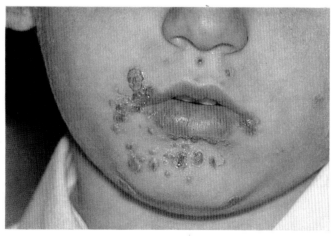

Fig. 71. Impetigo contagiosa streptogenes

It hardly needs to be emphasized that skin diseases due to cocci occur more often in children with chronic nutritional disturbances, and take a more serious course. Maceration (humidity and heat, desquamative nasal, oral, or anogenital inflammations), pediculosis capitis and scabies favor such manifestations. The same is observed in states of decreased immunity (syndrome of absent antibodies) as seen nowadays in patients who have been treated with cortisone or immune depressant drugs. Pyogenic foci of the skin can in turn occasionally give rise to involvement of internal organs, for example, the *impetigo nephritis*, which is not rare. This renal complication can be silent and may be discovered only upon routine urinalysis; on the other hand, renal involvement may become evident in a stormy clinical course with edema and hematuria.

Among the many pyodermas, "impetigo noncontagiosa staphylogenes" of ERASMUS WILSON (1850) and MAX BOCKHARDT (1887) deserves attention; it presents a pinhead to small lentil-sized pustule, sometimes having a red halo. Sometimes this pyoderma represents a superficial folliculitis (impetigo Bockhardt) or, in infants, a periporitis. Sometimes it is located in the subcorneal layer without any connection to cutaneous appendages. At times the fine lanugo hair perforating the pustule is not visible.

The furuncle may sometimes develop from follicular impetigo (BOCKHARDT), but more frequently begins as an inflammatory nodule in the depth of the cutis; it represents inflammation of the hair follicle apparatus and its surroundings, and has a typical central necrotizing plug. The furuncle may on rare occasions follow a subacute course, with central viscous softening; this development is typical in the patient with endogenous eczema. In contrast to the solitary furuncle, conglomerate furuncles are called cribriform (sievelike) furuncles; if there is more extensive infiltration (which occurs chiefly on the nape) the term carbuncle is applied.

Morphologically and etiologically related to furuncles and furunculosis (which may have a constitutional basis such as diabetes) are the highly therapy-resistant abscesses of the eccrine sweat glands. LEWANDOWSKY aptly called this process *periporitis*. These abscesses occur as numerous bluish-red or brownish (before perforation) and above all torpid abscesses, which may, nevertheless, perforate spontaneously. They usually appear on the back of the scalp and neck, the buttocks, or the back. They are frequently accompanied by superficial pustulosis which, however, is almost always absent in the apocrine sweat gland abscesses (of the axillae and genitoanal region) in the adult.

Superficial pyodermas, which ordinarily comprise 70 per cent of all pyodermas in children, are, at the nursery age, mostly due to a superficial streptoderma and show thick honey or amber-colored crusts, as described by TILBURY FOX. The adult presents superficial staphylodermas, shallow, thin, lacquerlike, crusted vesicles with a tendency to residual pigmentation. Staphylodermas of this sort are apparently more prevalent in warm summer weather, whereas streptodermas occur more often in the autumn. If both types of cocci are found in a lesion, the clinical picture of honey-yellow crusts will prevail.

Bullous staphyloderma *(impetigo contagiosa staphylogenes)* may show increasing severity (pemphigus neonatorum), especially in infants. The palms and soles are spared. These areas are favored by pemphigus syphiliticus. A climax is reached in the so-called *dermatitis exfoliativa* (RITTER VON RITTERSHAIN, 1878). This acute and fulminant condition results in

42

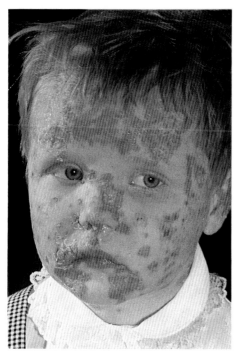

Fig. 72. Impetigo contagiosa streptogenes

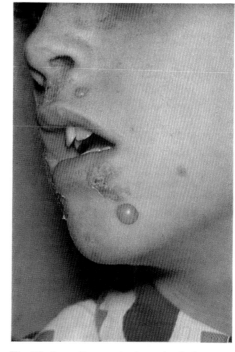

Fig. 73. Impetigo contagiosa staphylogenes

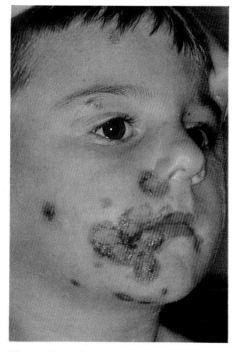

Fig. 74. Impetigo contagiosa staphylogenes
with thin crusts

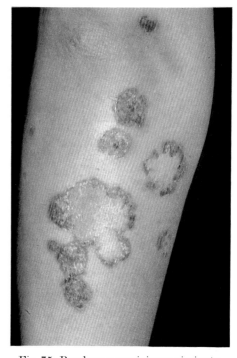

Fig. 75. Pyoderma serpiginosa circinata

43

rapid and extensive bullous exfoliation with characteristic residual patches that are eroded, erythematous, and moist. Epidermolysis with a positive Nikolsky sign may be the final result. The epidermis can be stripped off tangentially, as in exfoliative erythroderma, like the skin of a ripe peach. In adults this kind of superficial bullous staphyloderma has recently been called Lyell syndrome *(toxic epidermal necrolysis);* KORTING and HOLZMANN named it *epidermolysis acuta toxica.* In their opinion, however, in the adult this is the maximal variant of a toxic bullous epidermolytic exanthem. The staphylogenous variety prevails in infants and children.

Ecthyma simplex is an erosive ulcerous streptoderma of the epidermal-dermal layer. The disease has always been considered a "dirt" disease, caused by unfavorable hygienic conditions and minute traumas (stubble disease). *Ecthyma gangrenosum* is said to be caused by pseudomonas aeruginosa (bacterium pyocyaneum); ecthyma contagiosum (ORF) is a viral skin disease similar in appearance to paravaccinial milker's nodules.

Once in a while a superficial streptoderma may present with a bulla, the so-called *bulla rodens* (T. FOX and E. LESSER), or with a felon when located at the terminal phalanx of a finger.

Perlèche

JUSTIN LEMAISTRE (1896) still thought that a special "streptococcus plicatilis" was responsible for this erythema. Medical teaching today, however, considers the infected corner of the mouth as primarily a variation of streptococcal pyoderma, and only infrequently caused by other organisms. This would seem to be proved if adolescents (mostly male) simultaneously present a felon or retroauricular intertrigo. Should the condition be exceptionally stubborn one should look for underlying congenital fistulas of the corners of the mouth. Only in the adult will it be necessary to consider interlabial mycosis (candidiasis); the underlying cause may be lack of gastric secretion, iron deficiency (amenable to iron therapy), ariboflavinosis (for example, in diabetes mellitus), badly fitting dentures, and other causes.

Chronic vegetating pyodermas

Knowledge of chronic vegetating pyodermas such as *pyodermia chronica papillaris et exulcerans* (ZURHELLE and KLEIN) or *pyodermia ulcerosa serpiginosa* is important in differential diagnosis with tuberculosis cutis verrucosa, tubero-ulcerous syphilids and certain mycoses (sporomycosis and blastomycosis). Chronic vegetating pyodermas occur much less frequently in children than in adults. Spongy, edematous, verrucous or fistulous cutaneous changes frequently follow injuries. A wide spectrum of causative organisms is found (proteus vulgaris, pseudomonas aeruginosa; KORTING: streptococcus fecalis). Among other developments noted are autosensitization and embolic metastatic phenomena (such as syntropy with the same organism in ulcerative colitis and pyoderma gangrenosum), loss of tissue resistance, low gamma globulin, and many others. *Ecythyma gangrenosum* or *terebrans* (HALLOPEAU) affects malnourished, debilitated young children and only rarely adults with such conditions (KORTING and ADAM).

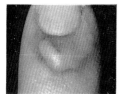

Fig. 76. Bullous
pyoderma of the
nail bed

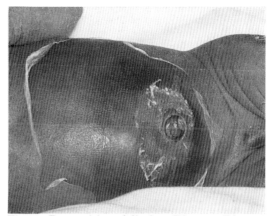

Fig. 77. Dermatitis exfoliativa (Ritter v. Rittershain)

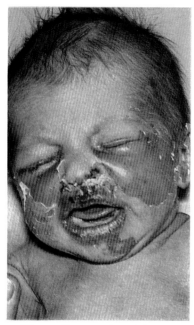

Fig. 78. Dermatitis exfoliativa
(Ritter v. Rittershain)

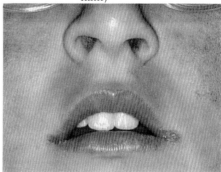

Fig. 80. Perlèche

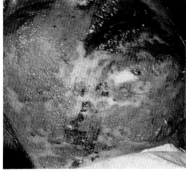

Fig. 79. Toxic epidermal necrolysis
(Lyell's disease)

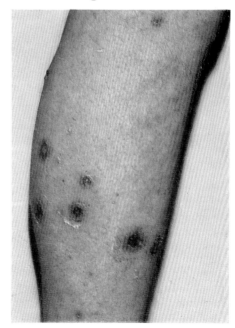

Fig. 81. Ecthyma simplex

45

Erysipelas

Erysipelas, formerly thought to be caused by a special "streptococcus erysipelatosus" (FEHLEISEN, 1882), occurs in the newborn and in children. Even in this age of antibiotics it still has a grave prognosis. Gangrenous erysipelas or facial erysipelas in the adult are also considered serious. As a rule, the primary eruption is accompanied initially by severe headache, nausea, and so forth. These signs may be absent in the young child. Furthermore, the edematous erythema and the sharp border may not be as pronounced in children as in adults. Erysipelas in children and infants, however, apparently tends to phlegmonous changes or even liquefaction. Portals of entry for the organisms are umbilical or circumcision wounds, piercing marks of the ear lobes, perlèche, rhagades in general, especially those of the ear canals and nose, and later in life toe-webs with preceding fungous infections. If there are no complications, erysipelas regresses in about one week; but because the antistreptolysin titer does not rise regularly, slowly developing recurrences may result in elephantiasis nostras and are not at all rare.

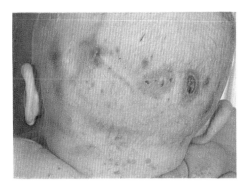

Fig. 82. Ecthyma terebrans or cachecticorum

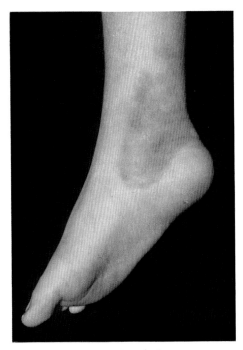

Fig. 83. Erysipelas

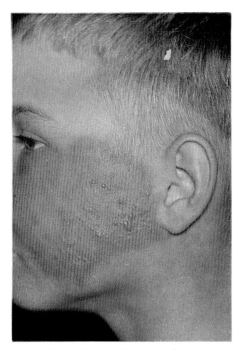

Fig. 84. Erysipelas vesiculosum

7. Chronic Infectious Diseases of the Skin

Tuberculosis cutis

In infants and young children tuberculous lesions of the skin and mucous membranes are relatively rare, with the exception of the tuberculous primary inoculation complex and miliary tuberculosis of the skin. The causative organism is Koch's bacillus, the sporeless, gram-positive Mycobacterium tuberculosis. Three main types have been cultured: typus humanus, bovinus, and avium. The appearance of the skin lesions differs according to an absent, changing, or hyperergic state of allergy, but it is also possible that it is somewhat dependent upon the peripheral blood supply, among other factors.

Tuberculous diseases of the skin *(primary inoculation complex, miliary tuberculosis, lupus vulgaris, scrofuloderma, tuberculosis verrucosa cutis, tuberculosis miliaris ulcerosa of the skin and mucous membranes, disseminated miliary lupus of the face)* are caused either by direct external infections, by contiguity with an infection reaching different layers of the skin, or finally by dissemination via the lymphatics or blood vessels. DARIER (1896) gave the name of *tuberculids* to specific microbids characterized by short duration and spontaneous involution and occurring in individuals with a high degree of immunity (thus the relative paucity of bacilli in the lesions!) in the late stage of generalization of tuberculosis by hematogenous dissemination. One distinguishes *lichen scrofulosorum, erythema induratum, and papulonecrotic tuberculid.*

Tuberculous primary inoculation complex of the skin and mucous membranes

A livid papule or pustule-like lesion which develops into a small shallow ulcer with many bacilli is observed almost exclusively in infants and young children who are in a state of anergy or still absent "allergic" response. Usually the face is affected, but in girls occasionally the vulval region (BRUUSGAARD) is involved. After a while the ulcer assumes a tuberculous appearance, showing a dirty base with undermined edges, and a fine, whitish, or in certain regions a somewhat keloidal scar results. Later, miliary papules, somewhat resembling lupus nodules, erupt perifocally. Such a picture may occasionally be seen after BCG inoculation, usually with enlargement of the nearest regional group of lymph nodes. Liquefaction and a subsequent tendency to calcification are characteristic.

Miliary disseminated tuberculosis of the skin

Tuberculosis cutis disseminata miliaris is practically restricted to infants and young children, but it is extremely rare today. It appears following a fulminant primary complex in the presence of miliary tuberculosis of the entire body, or in a phase of negative anergy after measles or whooping cough. The exanthem occasionally presents hemorrhagic, lichenoid, papular lesions which may show central necrosis. The exanthem is barely visible and resembles a miliary-lichenoid tuberculid resulting from generalization or a septic hemorrhagic exanthem of different origin.

Tuberculosis miliaris ulcerosa cutis et mucosae

Patients in a state of complete anergy but with florid open tuberculosis (that is, having a tuberculin-negative response) may develop before death an ascending tuberculosis through autoinoculation with highly infectious secretions, particularly those shed through the mouth and anus. Shallow, undermined, yellowish-gray necrotic ulcerations develop. These ulcerations are remarkably stationary and painless. This condition is usually seen around the age of 30 to 40; such instances have seldom been observed in children under 10.

Lupus miliaris disseminatus of the face (T. Fox, 1878)

This condition affects young men more often than women. There are varying phases of allergic response. First, the face, especially the midface including the upper eyelids and the upper lip, presents closely agminated disseminated hemispherical papules 3 to 4 mm. in diameter. The papules are light to bluish-red in color. They remain unchanged for months or years, and histologically reveal the most typical tuberculoid appearance of all forms of tuberculosis and tuberculids.

In contradistinction to lupus vulgaris, there is no confluence of the solitary nodules, but like the lupus nodules, these can be depressed with a blunt probe. They heal with the formation of a fine scar. Disseminated lupus vulgaris of the small nodular type also has to be considered in childhood. This form of tuberculosis would, however, eventuate in larger plaques, located more frequently on the trunk and the extremities than on the face.

Lupus vulgaris

This most common form of cutaneous tuberculosis, so named by T. Fox, was known as early as the early Middle Ages (Roger of Parma of the Medical School of Salerno, Italy); it was later described by Willan and Bateman. Contrary to initial belief, and according to investigations by Proppe and Wagner, lupus vulgaris does not occur more frequently in children and adolescents than in adults. Persons affected with lupus vulgaris have pulmonary tuberculosis ten times more often than people without the skin disease. The incidence of lupus vulgaris in patients with pulmonary tuberculosis is four times higher than in people with normal skin. In any case, patients with lupus or any other form of cutaneous tuberculosis should be examined thoroughly for the presence of extracutaneous tuberculous foci, such as those of the lungs, bones, or urinary tract; this means that the sputum, gastric washings, and smears from the larynx should be examined for the presence of tubercle bacilli. The threshold for tuberculin and the hemogram also should be determined, and a suspicious rise of evening temperature should be investigated further.

In 90 per cent of the cases lupus vulgaris starts on the midface with a small, penny-sized, intensely brownish-red or reddish-violet tumid papule, which on diascopic examination shows blanching, revealing the subepidermal, apple jelly-colored, soft infiltrate of the lupus nodule (Hutchinson). The soft, specific infiltrate is easily depressed with a blunt probe, or better with a fine stylet, which will painlessly sink into the tissue. This characteristic fria-

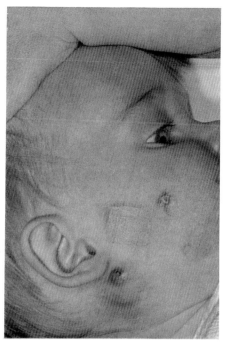

Fig. 85. Tuberculous primary complex

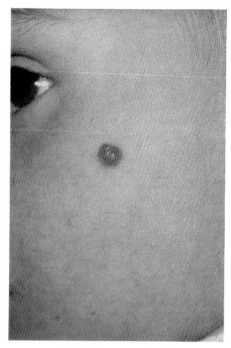

Fig. 86. Lupus vulgaris

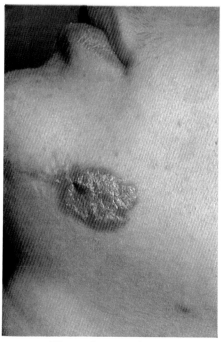

Fig. 87. Lupus vulgaris

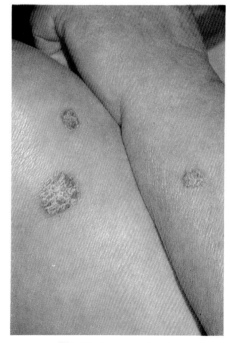

Fig. 88. Lupus vulgaris
"postexanthematicus"

bility demonstrated with the probe is better proof than seeing the "lupoid" infiltrate under diascopic diagnostic pressure, because residual pigmentations look similar; they cannot be made to disappear by diascopic pressure either. Lupus nodules may recur in healed, firmly atrophic areas, whereas lesions of tuberous tertiary syphilis (to be considered in differential diagnosis) do not recur in lesions healed with scarring. In children lupus vulgaris (as the so-called lupus postexanthematicus) appears secondary to acute infectious diseases such as measles or scarlet fever. The notorious mutilations, chiefly of the nose, and the lupus carcinoma (less frequently the lupus sarcoma) are, however, diseases of older people.

Tuberculosis verrucosa cutis (Riehl, Paltauf, 1886)

This form of tuberculosis is located chiefly on the fingers and hands. Histologically it differs from banal warts because of its perifocal, livid-red, leukocytic infiltration. It is the result of an exogenous superinfection in an individual who has previously become infected with tuberculosis and is in a normergic state of response.

This condition is observed in association with certain occupations (butchers, farmers, and veterinarians); its occurrence among medical students working in institutions of pathology is noteworthy.

Tuberculosis cutis colliquativa (scrofuloderma)

As in tuberculosis verrucosa cutis, there is a state of normergic response in scrofuloderma. The dermatosis shows lymphonodular and, less frequently, purely cutaneous-subcutaneous, gummatous infiltrates, which are matted together with the surrounding tissue over wide areas. There is a tendency to central liquefactive degeneration. Initially the dermatosis is skin-colored, but it soon turns into brown to bluish-red, painless infiltrations. In children these lesions may occur chiefly in the neck region below the mandible and in the sternocleidomastoid muscle; the scrofuloderma caused by hematogenous spread prefers a location on the chest or the back. (Among the mucous membrane lesions, scrofuloderma of the tongue should be mentioned.) Characteristic of the disease are "knitted" or funnel-like residual scars which last throughout life. In about every tenth case, lupus vulgaris will develop in the scar of scrofuloderma; MONCORPS, therefore, called scrofuloderma the "pacemaker of lupus."

The superstition surrounding the "scrofulous diathesis" is interesting from a historical point of view. Even ALIBERT (1768–1837), who first described mycosis fungoides, and DUPUYTREN (1778–1835) brought patients with scrofuloderma before the French king (1824) with the request that the diseased cervical lymph nodes be cured by being touched ("toucher les écrouelles") by the king.

Tuberculids

As already stated, the cause of such microbids, which slowly spread by developing into foci, was ascribed to the influence of tuberculo-toxins. These microbids were therefore separated from the processes produced by the bacilli themselves. Today tuberculids are generally

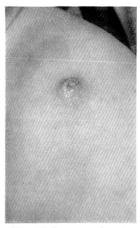

Fig. 89. Lupus vulgaris
following BCG
inoculation

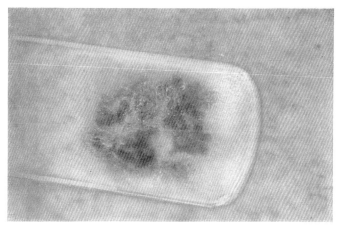

Fig. 90. Lupus vulgaris. Apple jelly-colored nodules (diascopic
examination)

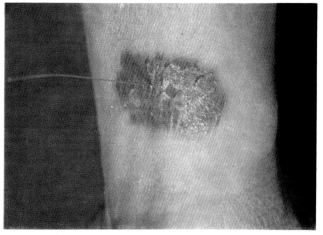

Fig. 91. Lupus vulgaris. Friability (probe test)

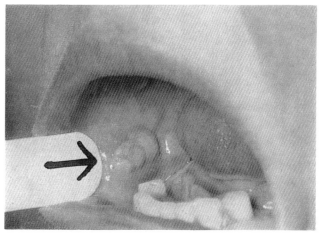

Fig. 92. Papillomatous lupus vulgaris of the oral mucosa

53

considered to be caused by hemobacillosis or emboli of bacilli stranded in the periphery, and because of considerable hyperergic response they dissolve quickly; it is therefore difficult to demonstrate mycobacteria in these lesions. Certain clinical entities such as tuberculids proper are differentiated according to their location in the skin and the amount and intensity of dissemination. Attempts have been made to destroy the concept of the tuberculids and to consider the papulonecrotic tuberculids as belonging to the group of arteriolitis hyperergica (RUITER), in a broader etiologic pathogenetic concept.

Lichen scrofulosorum

HEBRA (1860) first described a lichenoid form of tuberculids as "tetter of scrofulous individuals." Many minute, barely visible, yellow-red or skin-colored papules arranged in groups in an exanthematous eruption appear chiefly on the sides of the trunk. The lesions are follicular and occasionally acuminate. They show spinous excrescences, are papulo squamous (BOECK) or occasionally folliculo-eczematoid, or change (rarely) into pustules. HEBRA stressed the "scrofulous" overall picture: the simultaneous presence of lymphadenopathy, specific blepharoconjunctivitis, iridocyclitis, osseous tuberculosis and other signs. In differential diagnosis one has to consider lichenoid variations of other dermatoses, such as the mycoses and follicular keratoses – "spinulosism," lichen syphiliticus, and lichen planus acuminatus, including lichen nitidus.

Papulonecrotic tuberculid

These lesions are located deeper in the cutis and subcutis than the tuberculids mentioned above. They are more disseminated and found on circumscribed areas of the trunk, buttocks, and lower extremities. These papulopustular necrotic lesions may increase to the size of a hazel nut. They become soft, drain, and heal quickly with scar formation. In adolescence the lesions resemble acne, which gave rise to names (now obsolete) such as folliclis and acnitis. Lesions typically appear in successive crops, with a manifest dependence upon disturbances of the peripheral blood supply and the exogenous influence of cold. In infants and young children the similarity to miliary tuberculosis is striking. Cases before puberty however are extremely rare.

Erythema induratum

Common sites of erythema induratum are the flexor sides of the legs. Occasionally the lesions are located on the buttocks or arms. Compared to the papulonecrotic tuberculid, erythema induratum presents fewer single lesions. The lesions are situated in the deep cutis or subcutis and affect the vascular system in these deep layers of the skin. They are relatively stationary, only mildly tender, and develop in successive crops with bluish-red, platelike,

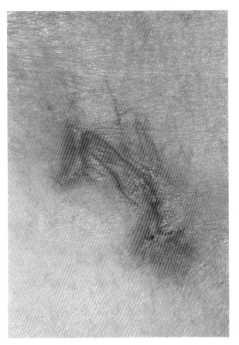

Fig. 93. Scrofuloderma

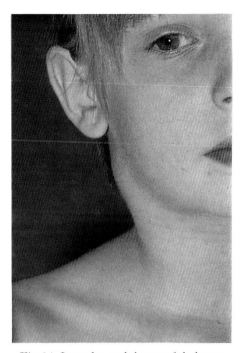

Fig. 94. Lympho-nodular scrofuloderma

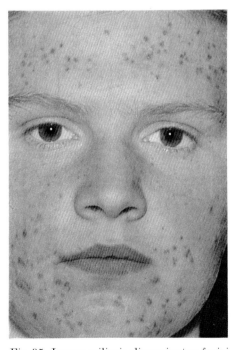

Fig. 95. Lupus miliaris disseminatus faciei

nodular or cordlike infiltrations which occasionally ulcerate (type HUTCHINSON). Bazin noted the preference of the disorder for the female sex. The disease occurs around puberty and the menopause, primarily in those young girls and older women who are sensitive to cold.

DARIER and ROUSSY (1904) described the *subcutaneous sarcoid;* its classification is controversial. Some authors consider it a deep form of erythema induratum or sarcoid; others regard it as lupus erythematosus profundus or the result of a lymphoreticular hyperplasia. Because of the location of the lesions in the deep cutaneous layers, erythema is absent; furthermore, similar nontender pea- to nut-sized infiltrates can occasionally be felt on the wall of the trunk.

BCG inoculation

The bacillus Calmette Guérin (BCG, 1921), originally a bovine type of organism, has, through mutation, been deprived of its virulence so that it no longer causes progressive tuberculosis in human beings. The present practice of intracutaneous inoculation with this bacillus results in a wheal. Two weeks later a papule appears, after two months reaching the size of a pea. The papule may show fluctuation. After another few weeks the lesion heals with formation of a scar.

Histologic examination initially shows tissue infiltrated by leukocytes and after a few weeks a florid specific granuloma, which differs from other tuberculous granulation tissue because of the deposition of Schaumann bodies and nonlipoid crystals.

The cutaneous manifestations which appear at the site of BCG inoculation may initially resemble a tuberculous primary complex. The lesion may later suggest lupus vulgaris (LOM-HOLT, 1946). According to KALKOFF, however, such an occurrence should be considered as a specific tissue response following an extreme quantitative increase of the inoculation mechanism, on the basis of a special host reaction. Moreover, in contrast to those of lupus vulgaris, these lesions heal by themselves. Lichen scrofulosorum, granuloma annulare, or erythema nodosum may infrequently develop as an indirect result of BCG inoculation.

Tuberculosis-like dermatoses due to Mycobacterium marinum or M. balnei (Swimming pool granuloma)

Two to four weeks after bathing in rivers or swimming pools, patients may present with short vermiform or glanderous shallow ulcerations grouped behind one another. The ulcerations develop at the site of minor cutaneous injuries and heal poorly. Preferred sites are the face, hands, elbows, and legs. Histologically, tuberculoid structure with special "fibrinoid" changes predominates. Infection with mycobacterium balnei heals without treatment within six months to a year. Whether the organism is seen microscopically or not, the material should be cultured.

Dermatoses whose causes are discussed in connection with tuberculosis

Erythema nodosum. This nodular erythema affects the deep vascular regions, the deep cutis, and the septa of the subcutaneous fat. Erythema nodosum presents red, later blue-red indu-

Fig. 96. Lichen scrofulosorum

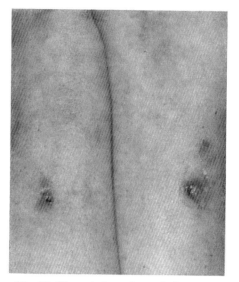

Fig. 97. Ulcerated erythema induratum

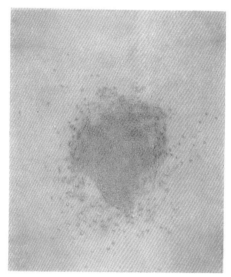

Fig. 98. Pustular reaction following
application of an ointment containing old
tuberculin (Moro reaction)

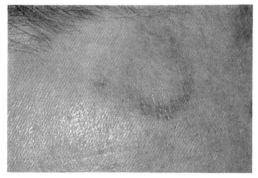

Fig. 99. Sarcoidosis (Boeck's disease). Annular
type

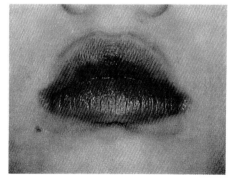

Fig. 100. Macrocheilia (Cheilitis
granulomatosa). Melkersson-Rosenthal
syndrome

rations, which are occasionally contusiform and rather flat. Lesions appear over the anterior aspects of the legs; they are less commonly seen on the thighs or extensor surfaces of the arms. In children, erythema nodosum represents a so-called "spontaneous Pirquet reaction."

Granuloma annulare. The etiology of this harmless necrobiosis is not known. In children and adolescents, who show a predilection for the disease, a tuberculous or rheumatic etiology has to be considered, because true papular tuberculids may have the same annular arrangement over bony prominences as granuloma annulare. The lesions of granuloma annulare are firm, nodular, somewhat pitted centrally, and nontender. In color they differ very little from the surrounding skin. They are arranged in characteristic bead-like rings and are located chiefly over the dorsa of the hands and feet, more rarely on the face (the eyelids and ears). As a rule, regression takes place without residual effect. Exanthematous generalization with predilection for light-exposed skin areas occurs infrequently.

Sarcoidosis. Intake and parenteral absorption of fundamentally different substances (quartz, beryllium, fungi, viruses, some helminths, flour dust, pollen of conifers, and similar compounds) may cause connective tissue cells to undergo metamorphosis into epitheloid cells. Diagnosis of sarcoidosis should therefore not be based exclusively on histology. The criteria for a diagnosis of genuine sarcoidosis (which is extremely rare in the first decade of life) are fulfilled only when characteristic granulomas, firmly encapsulated in connective tissue, occur in more than one organ (lymph nodes, liver, skeletal muscle, heart, and so forth). The disease may be of an acute, febrile, rheumatoid nature, or may progress slowly and asymptomatically. There are typical immunologic and chemical changes: a positive Nickerson-Kveim test, read after four to six weeks, a preponderantly negative tuberculin reaction, and occasional biochemical changes such as hyperproteinemia and hypercalcemia.

In spite of its systemic character the disease begins, as a rule, in the hilar region of the lungs, chiefly on the right side (KALKOFF). Pulmonary changes have been reported chiefly by KUZNITSKY and BITTORF, also by SCHAUMANN. They start as swellings of the hilar and paratracheal lymph nodes, and progress to pulmonary involvement in the form of lymphangitis reticularis. In addition small nodular miliary lesions or larger nodular infiltrates finally form diffuse widespread infiltrations. The osseous involvement already known to KREIBICH (1910) was described as osteitis "cystica" multiplex by JÜNGLING (1919). The parenchyma of the kidneys presents an epithelioid cell granulomatosis. The areas of the glomeruli become hyalinized and, most interestingly, nephrocalcinosis may develop. The central nervous system may become involved, resulting in diabetes insipidus. The Heerfordt syndrome (in analogy to the Mikulicz syndrome) shows involvement of the lacrimal and salivary glands. Its connection with BOECK's disease was recognized by TILLGREN in 1935, and is manifest in uveoparotid fever.

Although the cutaneous changes associated with sarcoidosis rarely occur in young children, theoretically, they may occur at any age. Such changes are observed chiefly in the second and fourth decades among females. Small and large papular to nodular, diffuse cutaneous and subcutaneous lesions are present. At first their color is reddish, later becoming more brown to bluish-red. An erythrodermic variant has not been definitely established. The face exhibits (rarely in children) the characteristic picture of *lupus pernio* (BESNIER, 1889) with extensive, infiltrating lesions (not to be confused with "chilblain" lupus, HUTCHINSON, which is a manifestation of lupus erythematosus) or the large nodular *angiolupoid Brocq-Pautrier.* Important in the child is the bluish-red infiltration of the ear lobes, which macroscopically cannot be easily differentiated from lymphocytoma or lymphatic leukemia. On diascopic examination the discrete lesions of cutaneous sarcoidosis look like dispersed pieces of dust

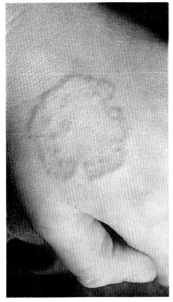

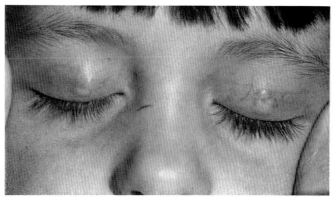

Fig. 102. Granuloma annulare; unusual location on upper eyelids

Fig. 101. Granuloma annulare

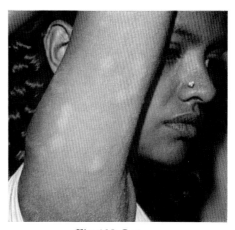

Fig. 103. Leprosy

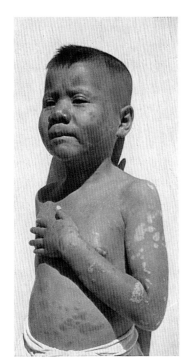

Fig. 104. Leprosy

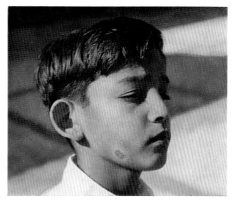

Fig. 105. Oriental sore
(Leishmaniasis cutis)

59

or specks (BOECK: sarcoid or miliary lupoid, 1889). They are arranged in circumscribed or exanthematous fashion. The lesions regress, leaving scars that are whitish or sometimes reddish at the periphery, and sometimes retracted as well. If the patches show preponderantly central involution, typically annular lesions may result.

Etiologically, and taking genetic factors into account, BOECK's disease has been considered to be a response of mesenchymatous tissue to multiple factors – a systemic reaction, or an atypical tuberculosis. Recent observations have shown that the serum of sarcoid patients does not contain antibodies against mycobacteriophages; the non-neutralized phages of tubercle bacilli are so altered that their presence cannot be proved by the usual methods (MANKIEWICZ, 1963).

Melkersson-Rosenthal Syndrome

Classified as being close to sarcoid is a syndrome characterized by scrotal tongue, episodes of facial paralysis, and pronounced granulomatous macrocheilia or cheilitis granulomatosa (MIESCHER), protruding edematous swelling of one or both lips with no color change. Initially transient but increasingly persistent manifestations have been occasionally observed on the buccal mucosa, the hard palate, and the periorbital region. In differential diagnosis one has to consider local elephantiasis following erysipelas, recurrent herpes simplex, or contact allergies.

The Ascher syndrome (1920) consists of blepharochalasis (dermatolysis palpebrarum) and variable changes of the upper lip (double lip, also glandular hyperplasia), sometimes associated with nonexophthalmic goiter.

Leprosy

In the entire world about 10 to 15 million people suffer from leprosy; in Europe the disease is rare, except for endemic foci in the southern part of the Mediterranean (Greece, Italy, and Spain). However, a few cases have been reported in Germany, where the disease was apparently contracted through contact with foreign workers (KALKOFF and HOLTZ). The infection with the Mycobacterium leprae (ARMAUER HANSEN, 1875) causes a not too highly contagious, chronic disease, which frequently begins in childhood when susceptible children acquire the disease in leprous quarters. Congenital transmission of leprosy seems to take place only in exceptional cases. On the other hand, a certain hereditary susceptibility seems necessary.

The clinical signs of leprosy vary greatly; characteristic is a close association of neurologic and cutaneous signs. The disease rarely spreads to the internal organs. After a long incubation period (usually about one year) and scarcely visible prodromal signs, depigmented, occasionally brownish-red plaques, and (much less frequently) papular or lichenoid patches develop. Characteristically, palpable thickening of some nerves (the ulnar and the auricularis magnus nerves) follows, with a tendency to abscess formation or calcification. In contrast to such symptom-poor beginnings, fully developed leprous changes are more distinct. The two main types are the highly infectious malignant *lepromatous form* (nodular lepromas of the ear lobes, supraorbital region, and nose, and finally leonine facies, involvement of the testes, and gynecomastia) and the type formerly known as maculoanesthetic leprosy, now called *tuberculoid leprosy*.

60

One diagnostic aid is to test affected areas for response to "sharp or dull" or to "hot and cold. '
Less important is testing the focal sweat secretion or the reaction of the arrectores pilorum; the
latter methods, however, may be of diagnostic aid in children who cannot give answers to tests
for sensory disturbances. In addition to histologic examination, smears may be taken from the
nasal mucosa with cotton swabs and stained with ZIEHL-NEELSEN stain. The MITSUDA (1919,
lepromin) reaction is important for the evaluation of the state of immunity. A standard organ
extract is intracutaneously injected; after two to four days (early reading, type FERNANDEZ) or
later – after two to four weeks – a papule is visible. The lepromatous type of leprosy is lepromin-
negative; the tuberculoid form with its favorable prognosis gives a positive test. A BCG inoculation may not only result in a change of the negative tuberculin reaction to a positive one, but
will act in the same way with the lepromin reaction. This gives hope for therapy and prophylaxis.

Leishmaniasis of the skin (Oriental sore, Aleppo boil)

This infectious disease, seen primarily in the Mediterranean and the Middle East, is caused
by Leishmania tropica and is transmitted by the sandfly Phlebotomus. A dirty brown infiltrate, and frequently also a bluish red lesion breaking down in the center, appears weeks or
months later at the site of the sting, and suggests at first glance a chancriform pyoderma. The
initial lesion spreads in satellite fashion, via the lymphatics, changing into small (later large)
nodules or verrucous-papillomatous lesions. In instances of low resistance the lesions are ulce-
ro-serpiginous and finally assume a plaque-like aspect in the manner of lupus vulgaris or lupus erythematosus. The primary lesion heals in characteristic fashion with the formation of
a scar after about one year ("year boil"). When primary lesions last for a long time, "leishma-
nides," small nodular lesions, may develop. The organism is seen in smears or in sections
stained by the Giemsa method. Dogs or cats are sometimes important intermediary carriers.

8. Virus Diseases of the Skin

Variola vera (smallpox)

Even instances of suspected smallpox must be reported to the authorities. The disease shows a regularly cyclic course with an incubation period of eight to 14 days. (Isolation, however, should be extended to 18 days.) *Varioloid*, modified smallpox in vaccinated individuals, is a frequent source of infection for variola vera, but the incubation period is eight days. Smallpox is an acute infectious disease with a grave prognosis. The virus is transmitted by droplets, dust, or fleas. At the end of the incubation period generalization of the organism takes place and is accompanied by acute high fever and severe malaise (pain in the lower back, extremities, and testes). A preliminary uncharacteristic roseola-like or petechial scarlatiniform rash may be seen on the lower abdomen or femoral triangle. Signs of a distinct upper respiratory infection (pharyngitis) prevail. Three to four days later, the organotropic virus has become fixed. This stage is characterized by abatement of the high fever and development of the smallpox exanthem on the scalp, forehead, nose, upper lip, trunk, and extremities, including the palms and soles but with only slight involvement of axillary and genitocrural folds and noninvolvement of the pubic area. All initial lesions are millet-seed sized. Firm elastic papules appear in crops. Around the sixth day the lesions are transformed into vesicles and around the eighth day they show central depressions and turn into pustules. On the eleventh to twelfth days they dry up, leaving characteristic scars. From the fifth to sixth days they all simultaneously achieve the distinctly uniform end-stage, which means that those lesions which began at a later time apparently develop at a faster pace. The most densely aggregated lesions are observed on the face, the dorsa of the hands, and areas of pressure.

In *varicella*, or *chickenpox*, there is no initial fever and no uniformity of the individual lesions – the rash is described by O. Heubner as a navigational map of stars – and small vesicles resembling water droplets arise from macular and nonpapular lesions. The extremities are only slightly affected, if at all. In addition, the lesions of varicella show a red halo more often than those of variola. The latter are multilocular and have a thick cover, which explains the longer persistence of the lesions.

At the time of the suppuration, which is accompanied by fever, the patient is severely ill (coma, restlessness, and circulatory collapse). Septic complications (suppurative arthritis, lung abscesses, or other septic processes such as nephritis, myocarditis, orchitis, encephalitis) threaten around the fifteenth day. Distinctly ominous is the presence of purpura or the intense edematous coalescence of single lesions.

The diagnosis should not be made from the clinical picture alone but should be confirmed by laboratory studies and epidemiologic evidence. For these studies it is necessary to submit to the appropriate laboratories (1) a thin smear of the blisterous contents on a fat-free sterile slide covered with another slide, (2) a thick smear of the blister content, air-dried, and (3) 5 to 10 ml. venous blood (without citrate). The patient in whom smallpox is suspected must have been in a place where single cases or endemics occur, such as Africa, South America, or the Indian subcontinent.

Complications of smallpox vaccination

Abnormal reactions to vaccinations, appear as pronounced perifocal erythemas, vaccinia secondaria or serpiginosa, oras vaccination-ulceration with facultative regional lymphangitis and lymphadenitis. Sequelae of hematogenous spread of virus are vaccinia generalisata (lack of antibodies ?) and postvaccinial eruptions of morbilloid, scarlatiniform, pityriasis rosea-like character, or those eruptions resembling a polymorphic erythema. Less frequently, purpuric, exfoliative, or nodular reactions occur. We speak of inoculation vaccinia if – analogous to secondary vaccinia in the vaccinated person – vaccinia is transmitted to another nonvaccinated person or to one who is no longer immune.

Equally grave as generalized vaccinia prognostically is *eczema vaccinatum*, which clinically may resemble genuine smallpox, with a fatality rate up to 30 per cent. It arises chiefly on a chronic eczema of a patient with neurodermatitis or atopic eczema. Such patients, therefore, should never be vaccinated, even if only mild cutaneous changes are present or doses of cortisone have rendered the patient free from manifestations.

NASEMANN published the following guidelines for permitting vaccination of patients with eczema:
1. Healing of the eczema by intensive treatment; if necessary, in a hospital.
2. Subcutaneous prevaccination with vaccinia antigen (manufactured by Behringwerke, Germany) [only in persons never vaccinated before].
3. Vaccination one week later – preferably with sterile egg membrane vaccine. Careful covering of the vaccination site. Continuous treatment of healed parts of the eczema with mild ointment.
4. Continuous observation.
5. In case of recurrent eczema before the vaccination reaction has subsided, immediate hospitalization and doses of vaccine-hyperimmune serum.

In *eczema vaccinatum* (as in smallpox) after an incubation period of five to 12 days, persistent, multinuclear, centrally umbilicated bullae with a thick cover appear, chiefly on the face. Light-exposed areas are favored. The lesions are multiplied by new crops but finally heal on about the fifth day with scar formation. Involvement of the oral mucosa often occurs.

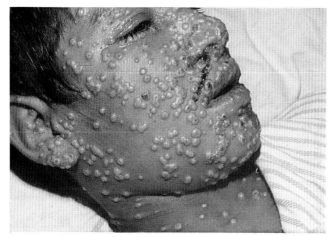

Fig. 106. Variola vera (smallpox)

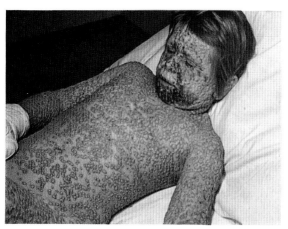

Fig. 107. Variola vera (smallpox)

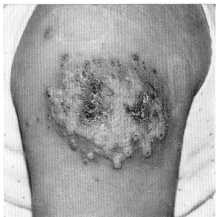

Fig. 108. Inoculation vaccinia

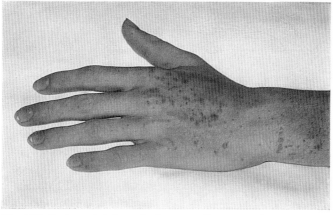

Fig. 109. Postvaccinial erysipelas spreading toward the left hand

In *eczema herpeticum* the herpes simplex virus rapidly spreads over the terrain of a manifest atopic eczema (cradle cap, neurodermatitis disseminata). The vesicles may be smaller than those of eczema vaccinatum, and unilocular. Oral changes are of an aphthoid character. Keratitis dendritica has been observed. The incubation period of eczema herpeticum, 75 per cent of which occurs in children, is only two to five days, which is distinctly shorter than that of eczema vaccinatum. Ten per cent of affected adults and 20 per cent of affected infants succumb to eczema herpeticum. Banal impetiginization of the so-called *varioliform pyoderma* type is easily differentiated from the two viral eczemas because severe constitutional signs are absent.

Patients infected with *cowpox* are almost exclusively milkers and farmers. Patients show a few anthrax or felon-like lesions which resemble smallpox. The lesions are complicated by lymphangitis.

The self-healing *milker's nodules* (paravaccinia nodules) are chiefly located on the fingers or hands of milkers. Other stigmata of this occupation are milker's tyloses or milker's granulomatous nodules, caused by cow hairs which have penetrated into the human skin.

Molluscum contagiosum (Bateman, 1817)

These clinically harmless infectious acanthomas are caused by a quadrangular virus which affects both sexes equally often and occurs in adolescents and children, occasionally even in infants. After an incubation period of two to three weeks or several months, pinhead to pea sized (giant mollusca) centrally umbilicated, semiglobular, elevated, slightly transparent or waxy tumors appear on the soft skin of the face, the eyelids, the neck, and the genitals. In an occasional shower of miliary lesions the central depression may be absent. With pressure from the side they discharge a firm but finely crumbled or granular white mass. There is mild bleeding. There are no symptoms other than occasional mild itching. The contagiosity is generally low. However, familial cases have been observed and a number of infections are known to have occurred in visitors to swimming pools.

Herpes simplex (herpes febrilis, cold sore)

Manifestations caused by the herpes simplex virus in the *primary* form occur chiefly in the young child up to about five years of age. They are accompanied by fever and general discomfort. The *secondary* type may not show many accompanying signs but is unpleasant because of its recurrent episodes. Predominantly adults, 20 to 40 years of age, are affected. They already possess specific antibodies. The most important form of the primary herpes simplex infection is *gingivostomatitis* or *aphthous stomatitis*, occurring in 70 per cent of infants and young children. It is accompanied by pronounced gingivitis, stomatitis with severe

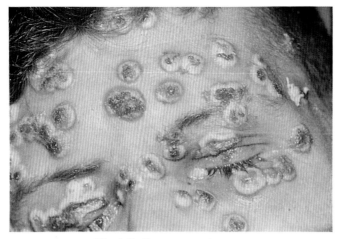

Fig. 110. Eczema vaccinatum

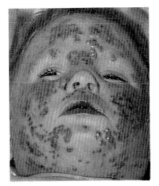

Fig. 111. Eczema herpeticum (disseminated herpes simplex; Kaposi's varicelliform eruption)

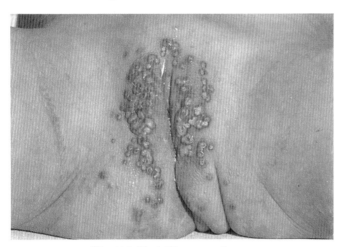

Fig. 112. Varioliform pyoderma

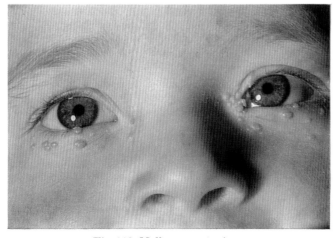

Fig. 113. Mollusca contagiosa

salivation, and conspicuous adenopathy. The initial lesion is an evanescent blister, which soon becomes eroded, covered with grayish-white matter and surrounded by a red halo. The lesion rarely ulcerates.

Aphthoid Pospischill – Feyrter is again a primary herpetic manifestation. It occurs as a secondary disorder in infants and young children who, not infrequently, after measles, whooping cough, and so forth, are in a negative anergic phase. Starting with originally isolated aphthoid lesions, the condition is characterized by wide, arciform, vegetating areas around the mouth, the nose, and also the vulva.

Much more common in older children and adolescents, however, is the secondary herpessimplex infection in the form of *herpes labialis*, or herpes simplex of other locations such as the buttocks or fingers. Characteristic are blisters grouped on slightly reddened skin or mucous membranes, and sometimes initiated by sensations of slight tension or itching. Recurrent attacks speak in favor of herpes simplex; concomitant neuralgic symptoms and segmental distribution suggest herpes zoster. (Decisive is the transmissibility of herpes simplex to a rabbit's cornea. GRÜTER.) From the time of puberty herpes progenitalis becomes more common. This is also the time of the beginning of the premenstrual herpes. This disorder is unpleasant because of its frequent recurrence. Herpes simplex concomitant with infections with diplococci (lobar pneumonia or epidemic cerebrospinal meningitis) and the so-called herpetic fever are relatively rare.

Herpes sepsis of the newborn, herpes embryopathia, herpetic keratoconjunctivitis, and herpetic meningoencephalitis should also be mentioned. Eczema herpeticum is discussed on page 66.

Recurrent herpes most probably develops through reactivation of "latent" virus in the tissue, or through reinfection from lacrimal and salivary glands.

Herpes zoster (shingles)

Occasionally, prodromal symptoms with moderately increased pre-eruptive temperatures for three to five days precede the sudden appearance of unilateral, bandlike, segmentally distributed groups of vesicles on a lightly red base, which may also for a short time be conspicuously edematous until the initially small, unilocular, clear vesicles develop.

Special forms are *hemorrhagic, necrotic,* or *gangrenous herpes zoster, generalized herpes zoster* (which may be varicella-like, predominantly in leukemias, reticuloendothelioses, carcinomatosis, or dysproteinemias), and *ophthalmic* and *otic herpes zoster.* Segments C_3 and C_4 are more frequently affected. These are the dermatomas of the phrenic nerve which, similar to Head's zones, may become irritated by processes in thoracic organs, via the splanchnic nerve, and also by abdominal disorders. Herpes zoster, therefore, represents a peripherally projected pathologic reaction on neurologic pathways and clinically signifies the second infection with the varicella virus in partially immune persons (DOWNIE). In children up to 10 years of age it comprises about 0.1 per cent of all cases of herpes zoster (NASEMANN). It is possible, however, that the incidence in children is actually higher, since there may be no generalized reaction and the course is much milder. There are no neuralgias, myalgias, pareses, or postherpetic pain. Children occasionally complain of mild itching or some tension in the affected area. Herpes zoster in the newborn is a still greater rarity.

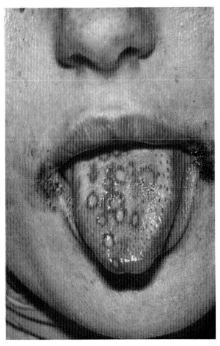

Fig. 114. Tongue with aphthous lesions

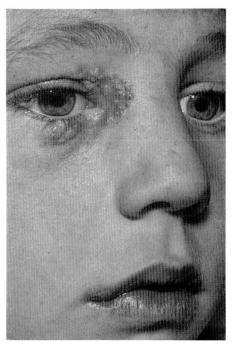

Fig. 116. Herpes simplex of right eyelids

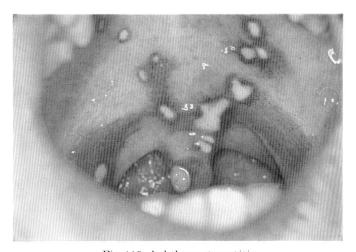

Fig. 115. Aphthous stomatitis

Varicella (chickenpox)

Varicella is highly contagious and is known over the whole world; it occasionally appears in epidemic or endemic form. Children up to about the tenth year, and less often newborns and adults, are affected. Two to three weeks after the infection mild general signs of lassitude, headache, and subfebrile temperature are noted. Infrequently an evanescent pre-exanthem of morbilliform or scarlatiniform character is seen. Distinct erythemas then appear on the chest. In the course of a few hours nodules and chiefly blisters, which are thin-walled, clear, and later become turbid, develop on these erythematous areas. New crops are the rule, so that various developmental stages are seen next to each other, and a relatively polymorphic picture exists. The individual sometimes umbilicated pustule of chickenpox lasts only a short time. It heals after one or two days, occasionally leaving a scar (on the face) or area of depigmentation. The patient remains contagious until the crusts fall off. The port of entry is the nasopharynx (droplet infection). Eventually, the trunk is most densely affected, although initially the head and face are favored. Not infrequently (although rarely in the infant) the oral cavity, and less frequently the genitals, show lentil-sized erythemas with central vesicles. Chickenpox is usually a mild disorder, but occasionally hemorrhagic or gangrenous transformations occur (beware of corticosteroids!). Other rare complications are pneumonia, corneal involvement, and central nervous system involvements.

Herpangina

This disorder occurs either together with other infectious diseases of childhood or as a disease entity per se with pronounced signs of a generalized illness (nausea, malaise, high fever, intestinal disorders, meningitis, and so forth). The clinical picture is characterized by grouped blisters on an erythematous base, located on both sides of the oral cavity, near the tonsils or uvula. The initial lesions look like frog's eggs or tapioca. After they have burst open they form small superficial grayish-white fibrinoid ulcerations, thus creating the picture of an ulcerative pharyngitis. Children between 1 and 7 years are affected – chiefly in late summer or early fall. This disorder is a manifestation of an infection with the Coxsackie virus. The prognosis is good.

Warts and condylomata acuminata

Warts, according to Jadassohn (1896), represent hyperkeratotic acanthomas and appear in four basic clinical types. Apparently, the same virus causes all four types; the differences among the types depend on the various specifically conditioned sites of the lesions.

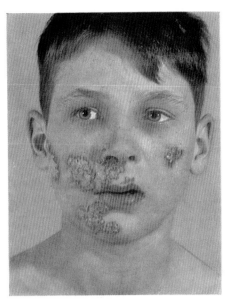

Fig. 117. Multilocular herpes simplex

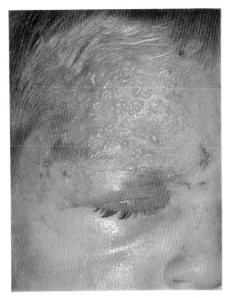

Fig. 118. Herpes zoster ophthalmicus

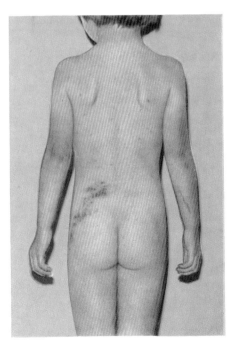

Fig. 119. Segmental and generalized herpes
zoster (varicelliform herpes zoster)

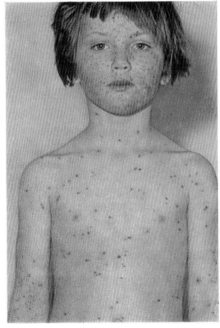

Fig. 120. Varicella (chickenpox)
resembling navigational chart of the stars

Verrucae vulgares, the common hard warts, are round or oval and also slightly polygonally outlined. Initially they are dark brown or grayish-yellow. With progressive keratinization they may even become black. In the beginning the surface is still smooth; soon, however, it becomes characteristically verrucous. Small, scattered, isomorphic *plane juvenile warts*, which barely protrude over the level of the surrounding skin, occur chiefly in children and adolescents, less frequently in adults. They may occur on any part of the body but favor exposed areas.

It is necessary to mention the following characteristic diagnostic signs of plane juvenile warts, since, as the name indicates, they are especially prevalent in children or adolescents and are frequently misdiagnosed or overlooked.

Plane warts never occur as solitary lesions. They appear in groups, or over wide areas, on the forehead, cheeks, chin, or the dorsa of the hands. They are pinhead-sized, round or polygonal, smooth, but most of all flat. They are occasionally slightly pruritic. They can be scratched off easily, which is followed by slight punctate, psoriasis-like bleeding.

Special clinical pictures of warts are seen when they occur on the eyelids, near the lips, or on the neck, as so-called *filiform warts*. *Mosaic warts* with their wall-like edge and finely contoured center are seen on the palm and the sole. *Subungual* and *periungual warts* are rather stubborn. Finally, the very tender *plantar warts*, because of pressure, do not rise above the surface of the surrounding skin of the sole. To the palpating finger they seem to be deeply imbedded, thorny pegs. Because they are often covered by callus, plantar warts are not infrequently misdiagnosed as pure hyperkeratoses or clavi. The skin-colored, rarely pigmented, plane juvenile warts, representing purely epidermal papules without papillomatosis, are easily scratched off, which contributes to their wide propagation. They may occasionally simulate lichen planus nodules or, especially on the hands, the lesions of Darier's disease.

The typical lesions of *epidermodysplasia verruciformis* develop on the dorsa of the hands and feet, usually before the tenth year of life. They are characterized by densely disseminated, preponderantly plane elements, which may become confluent, covering wide areas. Lesions comparable to verrucae vulgares are rare. Originally, this disorder was considered to be a genodermatosis, but at the present time the concept that we are dealing with a generalized form of disseminated warts (JABLONSKA and MILEWSKI) is gaining ground.

The last type of warts is *condylomata acuminata* (fig or moist venereal warts) which, in the form of pronounced papillomatous fibroepitheliomas, arise on areas of pronounced and chronic moisture (discharge) and are, therefore, located chiefly around the genital and anal openings. Their type of vegetation is compared to that of mulberries, cauliflower, or cockscombs. In condylomata acuminata spontaneous regression is observed less often than in other types of warts. Condylomata acuminata are quite rare in children. The favorite location is the genitals. The angles of the mouth or nose are affected only rarely.

On the basis of electron microscopic studies OVERBECK asserted in 1967 that the causative organism of condylomata acuminata is not identical with that of ordinary warts.

72

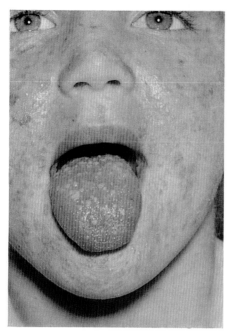

Fig. 121. Chickenpox lesions on the tongue

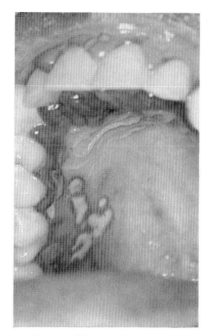

Fig. 122. Herpangina (due to coxsackie virus)

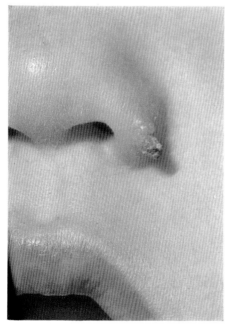

Fig. 124. Filiform wart

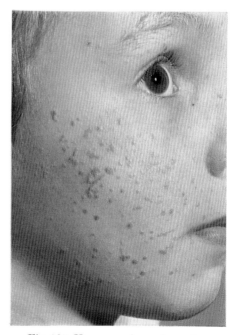

Fig. 125. Verrucae planae juveniles

Cat-scratch disease (virus-scratch lymphadenitis)

This benign inoculation lymphoreticulosis is probably caused by a virus related to that of lymphogranuloma venereum or psittacosis (MOLLARET: Miyagawanellosis lymphoreticularis). Since the original description by DEBRÉ et al. in 1950, about 1000 cases have been reported. A third of the patients are children below 10 years of age. About five to 15 days after a bite or scratch from a cat – which, by the way, is not diseased – or a thorn, a primary lesion (papule, vesicle, or pustule) forms at the inoculation site. This first manifestation is often overlooked. After an additional two to three weeks the regional lymph nodes become enlarged (primary complex, accompanied by mild malaise) and the original lesion is belatedly recognized as significant. The affected lymph nodes are not matted together. They may reach walnut size. There may be fever. In my own cases neither an exanthem nor an enlarged spleen was observed. As far as can be ascertained, this is a benign disorder.

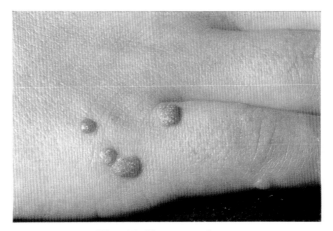

Fig. 123. Verrucae vulgares

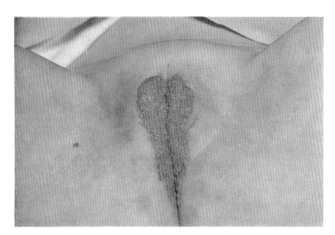

Fig. 126. Condylomata acuminata

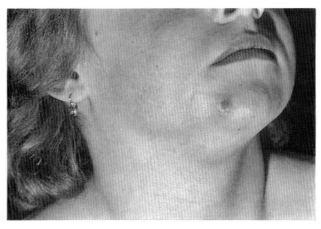

Fig. 127. Cat-scratch disease

9. Fungous Diseases of the Skin (Dermatomycoses)

Virchow coined the term "Dermatomykose" for a group of manifestations caused by fungi. They occur on the skin and mucous membranes, and can be classified according to their clinical appearance. It is difficult, however, to differentiate dermatomycoses morphologically and etiologically. (This must be done by culturing methods.) The historical concept of epidermophytosis has been replaced by "tinea," since Epidermophyton floccosum affects only the keratin of the epidermis and not the hair. In contrast, Epidermophyton Kauffmann-Wolf, now called Trichophyton mentagrophytes, and Trichophyton rubrum may affect the hair. This was demonstrated by the presence of folliculonodular mycogenic lesions on the legs of young girls and women. In analogy to the concept of tuberculids, we speak of mykids (Williams), dermatophytids, or id reactions. These eruptions are caused by toxins of fungi or by hematogenous spread of fungus elements themselves. Formerly, such eruptions were observed almost exclusively in children or adolescents and presented as a systemic disease (trichophytosis). Sometimes the eruption appeared after a diagnostic or therapeutic injection of trichophytin. Now we frequently see such id reactions in adults after treatment with penicillin. These are scarlatiniform, lichenoid, nodular, and rarely erythema multiforme-like secondary eruptions. Botanically, fungi are grouped as hyphomycetes, yeasts, and actinomycetes.

Favus*

Tinea favosa, a disease reportable in Germany and often occurring in several family members, is caused by Achorion or Trichophyton Schönleini, Quinckeanum. This chronic disease of the scalp is characterized by sulfur-yellow, cup-shaped, convex follicular crusts (scutula) consisting of closely matted mycelia. Uncharacteristic seborrhoid lesions are infrequently observed. A typical odor of mouse urine (acetamide) is associated with this disease. Favus heals with a characteristic scarring alopecia. Although favus rarely begins after the fifteenth year of life, it does not disappear spontaneously after puberty, as does tinea capitis.

---

* Favus is extremely rare in the United States. *The translators.*

76

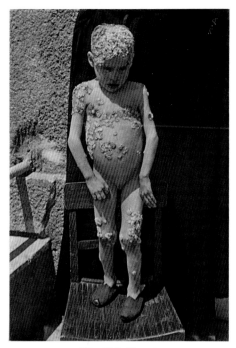

Fig. 128. Favus

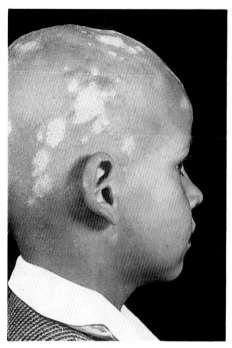

Fig. 129. Microsporosis

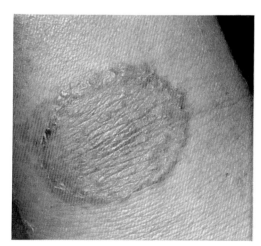

Fig. 130. Superficial trichophytosis

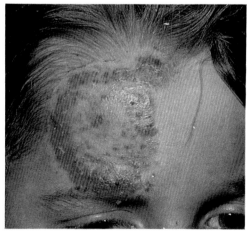

Fig. 131. Superficial trichophytosis

Microsporia (tinea capitis)

This fungous infection of the scalp (caused by Microsporum audouini), also reportable in Germany, is highly contagious, occurs exclusively in children, and may rapidly spread among pupils of the same class in school. Spontaneous cure is seen with the endocrine changes of puberty. The scalp of the adult is refractory to infection with tinea capitis. Children present with sharply outlined, round or oval, coin-sized grayish-white areas, with broken off, lusterless, short stumps of hair having a white sheath. These areas look as if they have been dusted with ashes or flour, or look like a badly cut field of hay. Red-haired individuals do not seem to be affected. The presence of the causative organism is easily confirmed under the microscope or by culture. For quick examination of large groups of children the fluorescence of affected areas of the scalp under Wood's light is of practical use; the affected hairs or scales show a bluish-green color.

Trichophytosis

This dermatomycosis occurs primarily among rural populations, in endemic or epidemic form. The fungi responsible for trichophytosis belong to the species Trichophyton (mentagrophytes, rubrum, and verrucosum in calves). We distinguish between deep inflammatory lesions with growth of spores and hyphae on the surface of the hair shaft, *ectothrix* (SABOURAUD), and superficial forms of trichophytosis with circular, map-like, peripherally exudative or seborrheic patches; in this type the spores develop inside the hair shaft itself *(endothrix)*. There are, however, transitions between the two types *(neoendothrix)*.

Deep trichophytosis occurs in children on the scalp, and has a honeycomb appearance (kerion Celsi). Frequently, areas of superficial trichophytosis of other parts of the skin with lanugo hair coexist. In the adult, trichophytosis occurs as a deep infection of the bearded region *(sycosis barbae)*, but since men have begun using their own shaving equipment, this infection is being seen less frequently. The initial lesion of superficial and deep trichophytosis is a small nodule or follicular pustule.

Mild circulatory impairment may predispose girls and young women to folliculo-nodular trichophytosis of the legs. This clinical form occurs in girls and young women almost exclusively.

Tinea (epidermophytosis)

This group comprises numerous mycoses which present various squamous, hyperkeratotic, and dyshydrotic features. They are caused by Trichophyton mentagrophytes, T. rubrum, and Epidermophyton floccosum. Occurring primarily on the hands and feet, they are acquired chiefly in later life. These mycoses represent a scourge of modern civilization. They may be contracted in bidets, bath houses, swimming pools, from walking on bathmats, and so forth.

HEBRA's *eczema marginatum* is now called *tinea of the groin or axilla;* it is the main manifestation of tinea corporis. Fungous infection of the nails occurs chiefly in adults. Paronychia is usually caused by monilia (candida). The following three saprophytic mycoses to be discussed occur in adolescents, but are never present in infants and only rarely in children.

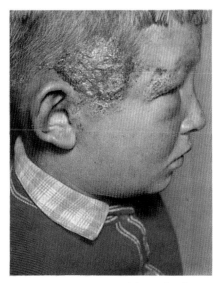

Fig. 132. Tinea capitis profunda

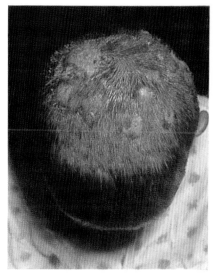

Fig. 133. Tinea capitis profunda
(Kerion Celsi)

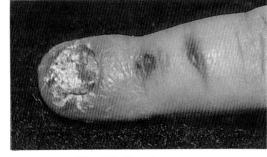

Fig. 135. Onychomycosis

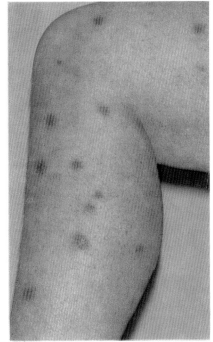

Fig. 134. Folliculo-nodular
trichophytosis of the leg

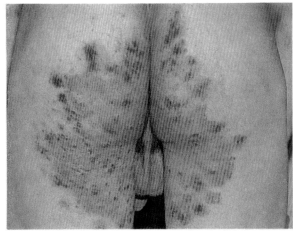

Fig. 136. Tinea corporis

Tinea versicolor

This superficial saprophytic fungus infection caused by Microsporon furfur, also known as Malassezia furfur, is found principally on the upper trunk in people who perspire profusely. Characteristic are irregular circinate or "geographically" confluent, yellow to brown scaling patches. Gentle scratching yields scrapings containing the fungi.

Tinea versicolor alba occurs on sun-exposed skin. The scales act as a light filter, preventing ultraviolet pigmentation of the infected areas.

Erythrasma

Adult males may present with irregularly outlined, faintly scaly, reddish brown patches on the upper inner thighs, next to the scrotum, but without involving it. Infrequently, the axillae may be affected. Wood's light reveals a reddish fluorescence. The causative organism, once thought to be Microsporon minutissimum or Nocardia minutissima, is now believed to be Corynebacterium (SARKARNY). The organism is sensitive to erythromycin. The affected areas present irregularly outlined, slightly scaling reddish-brown spots.

Trichomycosis axillaris

This tricho-saprophytosis, which affects mainly the axillary hair, presents bright red, nitlike, nodular sheaths, composed of a jelly-like substance called palmella or zooglea. The causative organism is corynebacterium tenuis.

Candidiasis (thrush, moniliasis)

In the group of blastomycoses – the fungous diseases of the skin and mucous membranes caused by yeasts or yeast-like organisms – infection by the genus Candida is of prime importance. This type of infection is common in intertriginous areas and presents erythematous, pustular, erosive lesions. Monilial infections of the nails and nailbeds (onychomycosis, paronychia) may also be seen. Other manifestations are perlèche, vaginitis, and balanitis. Many monilial infections of the vulva and anus have resulted from treatment with various antibiotics. The perianal skin of infants shows intensely red, lacquer-like, sharply marginated areas of erythema with satellite lesions and loosely adherent scales at the periphery. The mucous membranes of infants or edentulous old men present scattered, easily removable, white to yellowish-white "spongelets" on an erythematous base. This condition was formerly known as thrush. In infants the spots may be mistaken for remnants of milk. The source of candidiasis of the skin in newborn infants is quite frequently the monilial vaginitis of the mother.

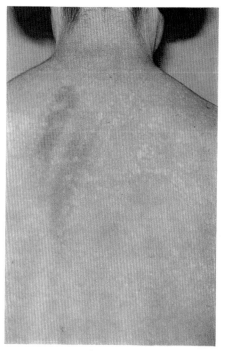

Fig. 137. Pityriasis versicolor alba

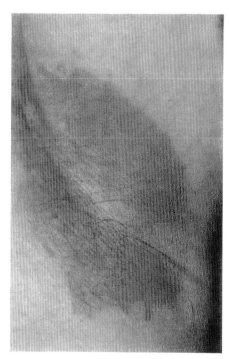

Fig. 138. Erythrasma

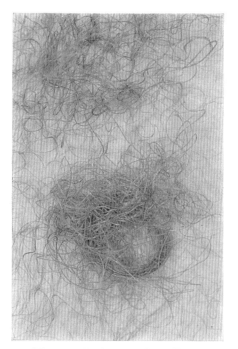

Fig. 139. Trichomycosis axillaris

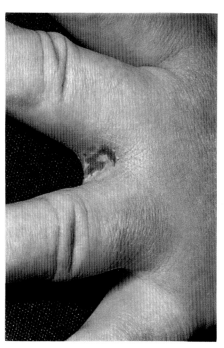

Fig. 140. Interdigital moniliasis (Erosia interdigitalis blastomycetica)

Actinomycosis

Three percent of all cases of actinomycosis are found in children. The disease is frequently seen in the cervicofacial region. The lesions may at first suggest scrofuloderma. True "lupus actinomycoticus" presents multiple subcutaneous, bluish-red, hard, infiltrated nodes. Much later these masses break down to form multiple fistulous tracts which discharge a purulent secretion containing "sulfur granules" (Drusen). The organism grows in culture on the Fortner plate, with microaerophils and other organisms consuming oxygen. The etiology of actinomycosis is not completely clear because there are numerous bacterial "satellite" organisms. An exception is Pseudomonas aeruginosa, which is conspicuously absent (Lentze). A constant companion of Actinomyces Israeli, however, is Actinobacillus actinomycetem comitans (Klinger, 1912).

A similar disease, nocardiosis, occurs in the tropics and subtropics. Tumorous, draining sinuses are characteristic. The causative organisms are the aerobic microorganisms discovered by Nocard in 1888. Other names are "mycetoma" and Madura foot.

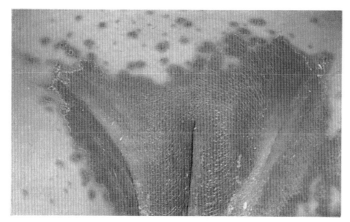

Fig. 141. Intertriginous moniliasis

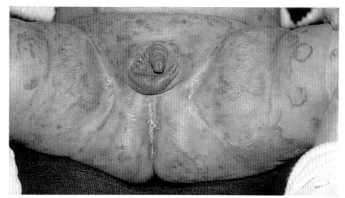

Fig. 142. Intertriginous moniliasis

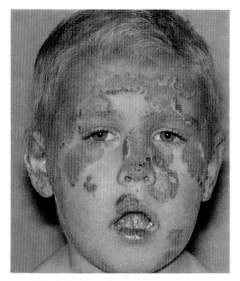

Fig. 143. Granulomatous moniliasis

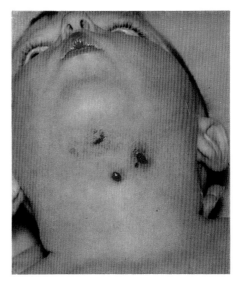

Fig. 144. Actinomycosis

10. Zoonoses

Scabies

Since the spring of 1966 scabies has occurred more frequently in Europe and the United States. It is caused by a mite, Acarus scabiei or Sarcoptes scabiei. After an incubation period of three to six weeks the female burrows into the horny layer of the skin, chiefly at night. It advances for a distance of a few millimeters, leaving characteristic ducts which contain debris and feces. The male, which is half the size of the female, is found only on the surface of the skin and dies after copulation. Children often present with ducts on the volar aspects of the hands and feet, on the glans penis, scrotum, anterior axillary folds, nipples, and umbilicus. The adult shows lesions on the buttocks. In the infant the face and neck are often affected; being nursed by a mother with scabies may cause such infestation. The blindly ending burrows caused by the mite can be made visible with fountain pen ink or ink pencils. They may be straight or angular. Blackish lines may appear, with a pearshaped "mite hill" at the anterior end. This hill represents a small vesicle containing the parasite, which can be lifted out with a needle or a scalpel held horizontally. Identification is then made with a magnifying lens. The burrows are often scratched open and after very little scratching they are easily visible. In addition there is a superimposed vesicular or papulovesicular eruption which, depending on personal hygiene, may be more or less pyodermic. Pruritus becomes increasingly fierce due to the warmth of the bed. This leads to scratching and excoriations, which in the adult may present as impetigo of the buttocks or in children as palmoplantar strophulus. A child who rubs the soles of the feet against each other while in bed should be examined for scabies. In children one has to watch for nephropathy induced by impetiginized scabies.

84

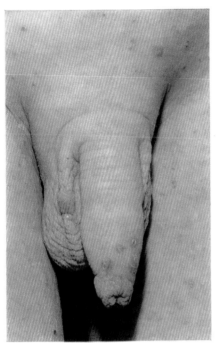

Fig. 145. Scabies

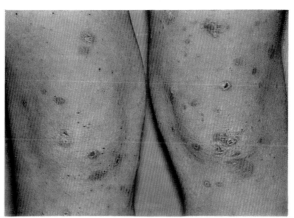

Fig. 147. Scabies

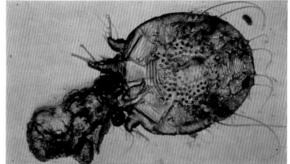

Fig. 148. Scabies mite

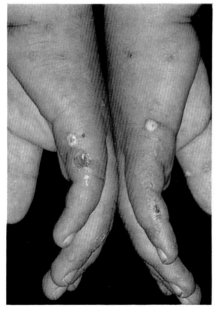

Fig. 146. Scabies

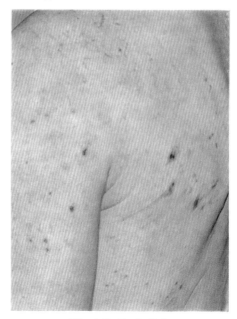

Fig. 149. Grain itch

Norwegian scabies, or *scabies crustosa*, is an infrequently seen variety presenting with severely scaling erythroderma. It affects retarded, cachectic, or apathetic patients. Either an allergic mechanism (eosinophilia) or "indolence of the skin" may be responsible. Hyperergic vascular changes and dysproteinemia may also be present.

Epidemics have shown again that in addition to human scabies, animal mites from mangy horses, dogs, cats, birds (Dermanyssus avium) or dead animals (game) can infect man. The bite causes severely pruritic papular lesions, especially at contact sites when tightly fitting pieces of clothing are worn. These mites live for only a few days or weeks on the skin and do not dig burrows, which permits spontaneous cure. Burrows are also absent when mites living in foodstuffs (dried fruits, tobacco leaves, cheese, and so forth) cause scabies-like eruptions, chiefly in food handlers. These manifestations can hardly be expected in children who are more likely to be affected by mites living in hay (leptus or trombicula autumnalis). These mites live for a short time on small circumscribed areas of woodland or bushes. *Grain or barley itch* is caused by the bite of a mite called Pediculoides ventricosus; it manifests itself as an urticarial erythematous or micropapulo-vesicular exanthem at sites of closely fitting wearing apparel.

The bites of ticks (Ixodes ricinus) which are brushed off branches in woody or scrubby territory are hardly felt, but the ticks adhere firmly to the skin. They become engorged with blood and assume a bluish-black color. They must not be torn off because the heads may remain in the skin. A good method for removing them is to first suffocate them with oil, petroleum, or vaseline. Cutaneous reactions following tick bites are discussed in connection with erythema migrans, lymphocytoma, and acrodermatitis chronica atrophicans.

Pediculosis

The head louse, shorter than the body louse by one posterior abdominal ring, nestles in the thick hair of women and children. It glues its eggs (nits), covered by a firm layer of chitin, to the proximal part of the hairs. The nits grow out with the hair. In contrast to the banal scales of seborrhea, the nits can be combed out only with a fine comb after preliminary treatment with vinegar. The secretion of the salivary glands of the sucking lice causes mild pruritus. Finally, through secondary infection due to scratching, there may result the nowadays rare picture of the matted, foul smelling "Polish plait" (plica polonica) with cervical lymphadenopathy. Along with the lymphadenitis one can frequently observe an eczematous blepharoconjunctivitis with phlyctenae.

Pediculosis corporis, or the presence of lice on the body and in clothing, has been observed in the last few years only in isolated cases among itinerants or vagrants without fixed residences and hardly ever in children. The adults present vagabonds' or vagrants' skin, resembling lymphogranulomatosis, senile pruritus, or prurigo Duhring. Acute pediculosis does not present excoriated melanoderma but a moderately urticarial or papular exanthema. The lice themselves are present on the skin only when feeding; they can be found in the seams of clothing (collars and sleeves).

Lately, cases of *pediculosis pubis* have been seen occasionally in children. The pale brown lice stay flat and scutiform and are motionlessly anchored either to the skin or to a hair. In children they can be found on the eyelashes and eyebrows, and occasionally on the scalp. The parasites prefer the sites of the apocrine glands; on the eyelids these are known as

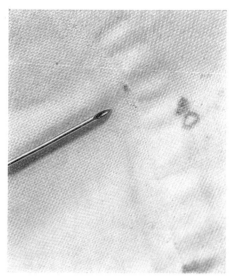

Fig. 150. Phthirius corporis (body louse)

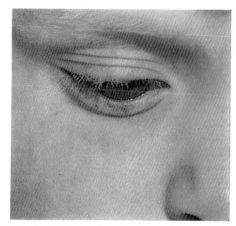

Fig. 151. Infestation of the eyelashes with pubic lice

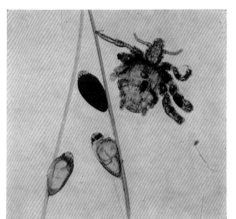

Fig. 152. Pubic louse with nits

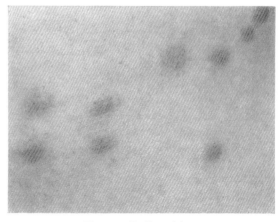

Fig. 153. Bedbug bites

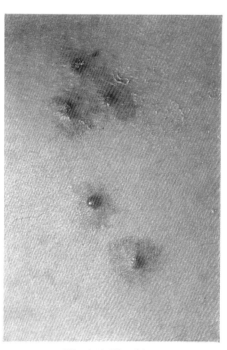

Fig. 154. Flea bites

Moll's ciliary glands. Bluish patches, the so-called tâches bleues (maculae caeruleae) are often seen. The bite of the parasite leads to the formation of degenerative products of hemoglobin. Because of the absence of severe pruritus there are no scratch effects.

Cimicosis

The ubiquitous, photophobic bedbug (Cimex lectularius) is yellowish brown in color, becoming somewhat darker after ingestion of blood. In the daytime it hides behind wall-paper, electric fuses, or in the joints of beds. At night the bedbug crawls over the exposed skin, and may even drop on the sleeper from the ceiling. The bite causes an urticarial lesion about 1.0 cm. in diameter. Whether exposed or unexposed, the skin over the joints, parti-cularly the hips, knees, or shoulders, is preferred. The linear distribution of urticarial macules following each other like footprints is typical. A hemorrhagic point is quite frequently visible at the site of the bite. If there is a special allergic response, bullae may appear; with decreasing sensitivity prurigo papules may develop. Finally, with increasing tolerance, papules may fail to appear. Bedbugs give off a certain odor from an oily body secretion.

Bee, wasp, and hornet bites (hymenopteriasis)

In susceptible individuals, especially children, bites by bees, wasps, or hornets cause extensive bluish-red swellings, which may occasionally last for days. The single lesion frequently shows a hemorrhagic point at the site of the bite. Pronounced swelling develops on the eyelids, the vermilion border of the lips, and the oral mucosa. According to the individual's disposition or his state of sensitivity, circulatory disturbances or systemic signs (sense of oppression, shortness of breath, diarrhea, asthma-like complaints) may appear. Multiple bites, chiefly those of young insects, are dangerous because of their cumulative effect. Laryngeal edema is especially threatening, as with urticaria in general.

Flea bites (pulicosis)

The flea is also photophobic. There are several varieties of fleas in the animal kingdom. The flea of the rat is responsible for plague. The bite of the flea and the secretion released with it, are highly irritating, causing an intensely painful itch which lasts for a long time. Light red, grouped macules with focal petechiae (purpura pulicosa) develop. The reaction to the sting varies greatly from one individual to another. Children in particular may show bullae. These may result in papular urticaria (strophulus infantum) which may also be caused by bites of other parasites.

88

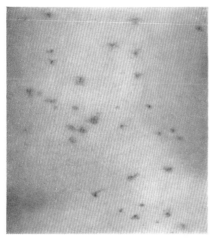

Fig. 155. Mosquito bites

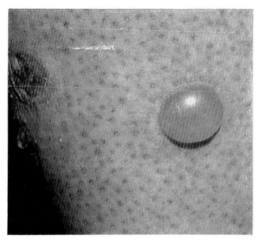

Fig. 156. Bullous reaction to mosquito bite

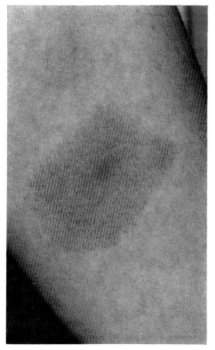

Fig. 157. Reaction to tick bite
(beginning erythema migrans)

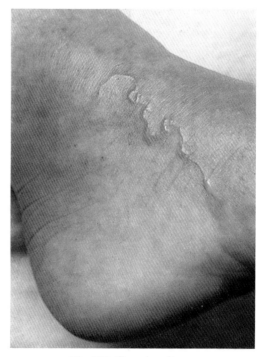

Fig. 158. Creeping disease

Mosquito bites (culicosis)

Mosquito bites give the same immediate pruritic reaction as the bites of other parasites, and in children they cause papular urticaria (lichen urticatus). On the legs, bullous lesions may simulate pemphigus (culicosis bullosa).

Caterpillar dermatitis (lepidopteriasis)

About 30 minutes after contact with the fine hairs of caterpillars, an urticarial reaction begins which may sometimes last for weeks. The reaction is occasionally associated with systemic reactions such as nausea and even albuminuria. The fine hairs of the caterpillar have the toxic effect. Local and general reactions are more pronounced if a caterpillar is squashed on the skin while being wiped off, since this leads to cutaneous contact with many more hairs.

Creeping eruption (myiasis linearis migrans)*

Creeping eruption, with its characteristic zig-zag figures, is caused by the larvae of several flies, chiefly the horsefly. Preferred sites are the feet, and less frequently the hands and buttocks of children who walk barefooted on a beach or play in the sand. Again, there is a tendency for nocturnal pruritus because at this time the "mole of the skin" is burrowing. There is also a so-called "ophthalmomyiasis." Larvae are found in eyelids, conjunctivae, the lacrimal appendages, and occasionally inside the eye. This results in a violent conjunctivitis, "tumors" of the eyelids, and serous iritis. This ocular involvement is seen chiefly in the tropics but has been observed in children in the region of the North Sea and the Baltic.

Jellyfish eruption

Stepping on the spike of a jellyfish at a beach, or merely coming into contact with its tentacles, causes gelatinous, later necrotizing or granulomatous cutaneous reactions.

Cercaria dermatitis (schistosomiasis)

Schistosomes are dropped into fresh water lakes in the feces of birds and develop to mature cercariae. These schistosomes cause heavy pruritus followed by small papulo urticarial lesions and later a widespread dermatitis unless the skin is rubbed with towels after bathing in the

---

* The creeping eruption (KIRBY-SMITH) is common in the southern United States and Puerto Rico. It is caused by the larvae of Ancylostoma braziliense, a parasite living in the intestines of dogs and cats. When their feces, containing the larvae, are deposited on an ocean beach above the high tide line bathers may be infected. When deposited under houses, they cause plumber's itch. *The translators.*

lake. Re-exposure may sensitize the individual, thereby increasing the severity of the erup-tion. This bather's rash has been observed on Lake Zürich, Lake Constance, and lakes in Germany.*

Skin manifestations of infestation with nematodes

In young children oxyuris vermicularis frequently causes perianal pruritus, dermatitis, vulvovaginitis, and less frequently chronic urticaria. The latter, in conjunction with marked eosinophilia, eosinophilic infiltrations of the lungs, or asthma, may be due to worm infesta-tion with Ascaris lumbricoides, pinworms, or trichuris trichiura, the thread- or whipworm.

---

  * In Puerto Rico, snails living in the fresh water lakes are the intermediary hosts. They carry the far more dangerous schistosoma haematobium, which may cause severe internal disorders. *The translators.*

11. Congenital Abnormalities of the Skin

Congenital abnormalities represent either considerable (malformations) or mild morphologic deviations from the normal. They lie outside the range of normal variation, and, if compatible with life, occur in about 0.5 per cent of the general population.

Anhidrosis hypotrichotica (Congenital anhidrotic ectodermal defect)

This ectodermal polydysplasia is characterized by hypohidrosis, hypotrichosis, and oligodontia. Clinically, these stigmata resemble those of congenital syphilis (frontal bosses, pronounced glabella, and small projecting ears ("ears of a satyr"). Complete absence of teeth is only rarely encountered. As a rule oligodontia is present. The absence of sweat glands causes disturbances of the thermoregulating mechanism (rising body temperature from increased physical effort). Not infrequently the breasts are malformed (hypomastia or aplasia, or polythelia). There may be a strong tendency toward markedly keratinized follicular channels, which assume the aspect of papular elevations (hyperacanthotic, rudimentary follicular funnels), seen chiefly on the cheeks or the temples.

In the minor type, the so-called hidrotic ectodermal defect, hairs and nails may be hypoplastic, but the sweat glands are normal.

Aplasia cutis congenita circumscripta

The newborn may show congenital hypoplasia of the skin. In later life, the defect, if present on the scalp, presents only with an atrophic lesion with alopecia. As a rule, changes are multiple. The individual lesion is usually not larger than 2 to 3 cm. in diameter. Favorite sites are the neighborhood of the small fontanelles, and the occiput on both sides of the midline. The defects have been blamed on early embryonal developmental disturbances, amniotic adhesions, or local intrauterine trauma. They have also been considered as the final stage of healed intrauterine epidermolysis bullosa.

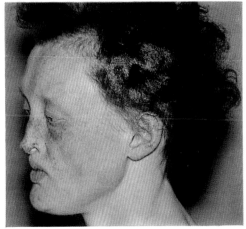

Fig. 159. Ectodermal dysplasia (typical facies)

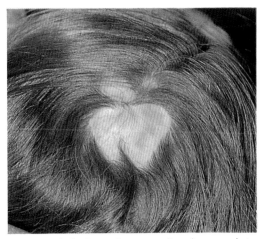

Fig. 160. Aplasia cutis congenita circumscripta

Fig. 161. Pachyonychia congenita

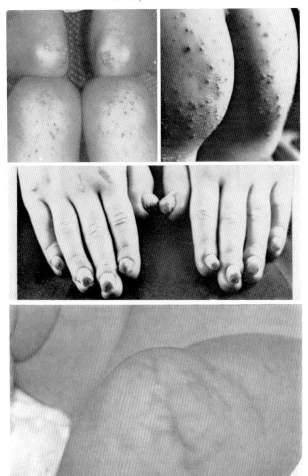

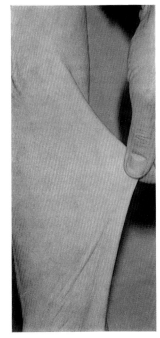

Fig. 163. Cutis laxa (Ehlers-Danlos syndrome). Cutis hyperelastica.

Fig. 162. Cutis marmorata teleangiectatica congenita

Pachyonychia congenita

This generalized dysplasia (JADASSOHN and LEWANDOWSKY, 1906) exhibits congenital polykeratosis with pachyonychia (extremely hard, compact horny nail substance), acneiform follicular hyperkeratoses over the elbows, knees, buttocks, or shoulder blades, palmoplantar keratoses, and finally leukokeratoses of the oral mucosa (occasionally hoarseness results from leukoplakia of the vocal cords).

Dyskeratosis congenita (ZINSSER, 1906), is discussed in connection with poikilodermal dysplasias.

Cutis marmorata telangiectatica congenita

In this rare, cutaneous, congenital anomaly, angiectasis of the vessels occurs. Vessels of large caliber are chiefly affected. The skin shows reticular, lattice-like livedo racemosa, arranged in figures or stripes. Around the tenth year of life the changes usually regress; this may bear some relation to the increase in subcutaneous fat tissue.

Progeria Hutchinson-Gilford

This disorder is characterized by dwarfism, acromicria, and a decidedly senile looking, tight atrophy of the skin and subcutaneous tissue. Other important signs are hypertonia, calcifications, thrombosis of the larger vessels, and premature arteriosclerosis, which involves the coronary vessels and the aorta, resulting in shortened life expectancy for affected individuals.

Familial *acrogeria* (GOTTRON, 1940) represents a minor type of the Hutchinson-Gilford anomaly. It is noteworthy that here, as in other congenital poikilodermas, there is a tendency to anomalies of keratinization or verrucous, ectodermal, peripheral changes such as elastosis serpiginosa (LUTZ-MIESCHER).

Cutis laxa (Ehlers-Danlos syndrome)

The fully developed picture of abnormal fragility of the skin and hyperextensibility of the joints and skin has not often been observed. The unusual vulnerability of the outer integument results in subcutaneous hematomas or gaping elliptical wounds following even mild

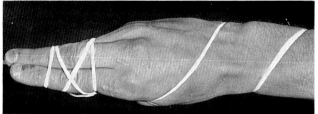

Fig. 164. Cutis laxa. The palmar arch can be abnormally squeezed

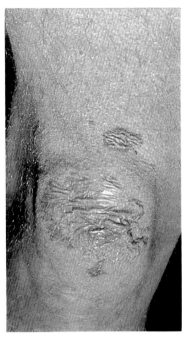

Fig. 165. Cutis laxa (characteristic redundant scars)

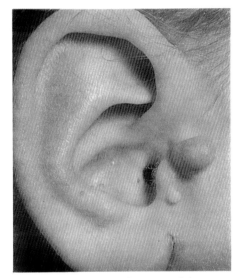

Fig. 166. Auricular appendages

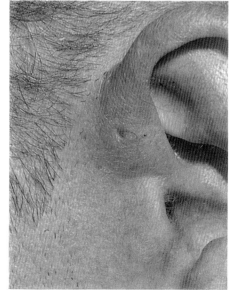

Fig. 167. Congenital aural fistula

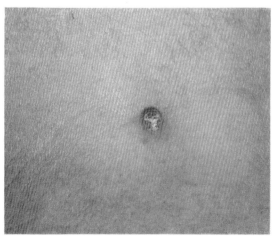

Fig. 168. Midline fistula of neck

trauma. Additional characteristic signs are cystic cavities in the underdeveloped sub-cutaneous fat layer, loose ligaments with hyperextensibility of the joints, and flaccid muscles in general. In children and adolescents mild hyperextensibility of the fingers, chiefly of the thumbs, is found rather frequently, as well as subluxations and habitual luxations. Because it may be part of other congenital developmental disturbances, a monosymptomatic hyper-extensibility of the joints should not lead to the diagnosis of the Ehlers-Danlos syndrome unless familial involvement can be determined. It is assumed that in most cases abnormal genetic factors lead to interference with the normal structure of collagen, resulting in connective tissue which is less well functioning.

Cysts, fistulas, pits, and similar anomalies

Ocular hypertelorism, observed by FAGGE as early as 1870 in association with ichthyosis vulgaris and named by GREIG in 1924, defines abnormal width between the eyes, with palpebral fissures similar to those seen in mongolism.

Auricular appendages do not represent supernumerary ears but rather chondrocutaneous hyperplasias, named branchiogenic cartilaginous nevi by SIEMENS and naevi cartilaginei by others. They are rarely associated with other branchiogenic anomalies, and represent some-times pedunculated tumors of pinhead to fingertip size in front of or behind the auricle. Tan spots are sometimes the sole abortive sign.

Congenital auricular fistulas are usually located in front of the tragus and in rare instances connect with the middle ear or pharynx. They either derive from the first branchial arch or are formed by the faulty merging of auricular tubercles. Stubborn eczemas or lupoid, lymphocytomatous reactions may be observed around these fistulas.

Congenital cysts and fistulas also occur on the nose and are usually located medially or para-medially on the dorsum of the nose. Occasionally, only a punctate depression is present.

Round or slit-like depressions may occur on the lips, either symmetrically or asymmetrically. Fistulas or dimples on the angles of the mouth are seen equally frequently. They may sustain a stubborn perlèche.

Besides primordial thyroglossal or branchiogenic fistulas, fistulas of the salivary glands and granulomatous fistulas may exist on the face. Others develop on the basis of ingrowing follicular openings or are the result of a foreign body trauma, actinomycosis, or tuberculosis, or appear as *odontogenous facial fistulas*.

Tonsilla linguae heterotopica symmetrica is an atavistic anomaly of the tongue. In most cases it is located on the posterior aspect of the side of the tongue. The anomaly shows gray to pinkish-red, about fingernail-sized, occasionally cerebriform, convolutional, and tumorous formations, which exhibit a lymphoepithelial structure histologically. If inflamed, it may cause pain comparable to that of a typical tonsillar sore throat. The *aberrant goiter* of the tongue is located on the base of the tongue (the foramen caecum). Much more frequent in this part of the tongue is *glossitis rhomboidea mediana*, described by BROCQ and PAUTRIER

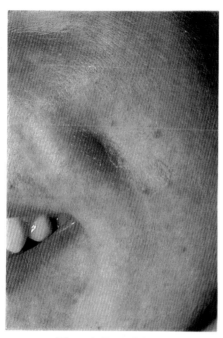

Fig. 169. Dental fistula

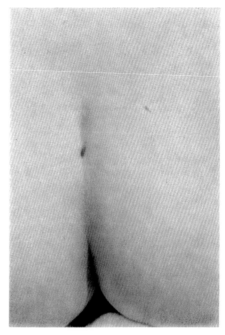

Fig. 170. Coccygeal fistula

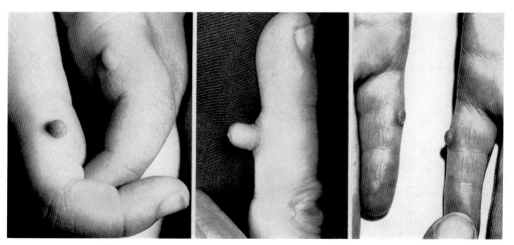

Fig. 171. Rudimentary polydactylia (supernumerary fingers)

in 1914. It represents a fissural angioma or hemolymphangioma because of a persistent tuberculum impar. Infiltrates of histiolymphoplasmocytes may cause transitory inflammations.

On the neck may be noted the rather infrequently occurring *medial* fistula colli and, more important, the *fistula colli congenitalis lateralis*, which presents an external opening at the anterior margin of the sternocleidomastoid muscle and may communicate with the pharynx.

Depressions on the acromion of the *shoulders* occur occasionally, becoming more or less clearly visible when the trunk is turned to the side.

Of greater practical significance, however, are sinus-like changes, which may give the impression of cysts, in the *sacrococcygeal* area. Located over the hiatus finalis sacralis, if severely inflamed, they may be misdiagnosed as furuncles or periproctic abscesses. This anomaly appears in small children only as *foveola coccygea* and becomes a distinct fistula after puberty following a secondary infection. On the other hand, only children show omphalomesenteric fistulas or cysts in the umbilical area.

Important among single malformations of the extremities is *polydactylism*, which is usually associated with various other stigmata (hypotrichosis, syndactilism or hypertelorism). Among *malformations of the fingers* doubling and, even more important, verrucous, tuftlike, or firm pedunculated *supernumerary fingers* should be mentioned. *Rudimentary polydactylia* may contain cartilaginous and nervous tissues.

Cutaneous anomalies in syndromes characterized by skeletal malformations

In various basic osseous disorders, such as osteogenesis imperfecta, the same almost stereotyped cutaneous signs are noted: the combination of pigmentary disturbances and hair anomalies, cutis laxa, anetoderma, and a nondeveloped venous network. Multiple lenticular dermatofibrosis is associated with osteopoikilosis (BUSCHKE and OLLENDORFF CURTH).

Dystrophic nails may call attention to the presence of the *nail-patella* or the Turner-Kieser *syndromes*, in which characteristic symmetric pelvic horns may be seen, as well as an hypoplastic anterior layer of the iris. My own studies (KORTING and GEBHARDT) have led to the classification of this disorder with the systemic mucopolysaccharidoses.

Children with *cretinism* exhibit cold, dry, or pasty skin. Those with *leprechaunism* have hyperpigmentation, hirsutism, congenital gynecomastia, and hypertrophy of the clitoris as well.

In addition to the known stigmata (epicanthal folds, a furrow of the fourth finger and isolated growth of the big toe), patients with mongolism (Down's syndrome) may exhibit ichthyosiform skin, acrocyanosis, cutis marmorata et laxa, a chronic permanent vasomotoric redness in butterfly distribution, follicular acneiform nodules, syringomas, and lingua and cheilitis "scrotalis." Not infrequently, multiple patchy areas of alopecia are seen on the neck. The posterior hairline is low (KORTING and HOLZMANN).

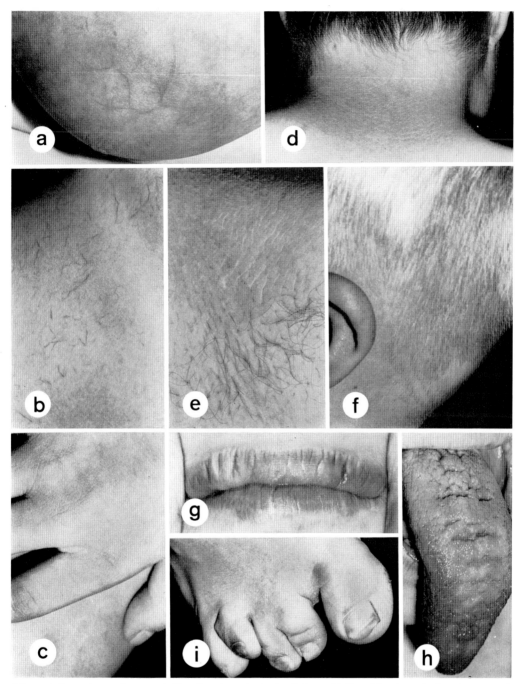

Fig. 173. Down's syndrome. a) Fine livedo reticularis of chest. b) Ramification of telangiectases of shoulder girdle. c) Cutis marmorata with finely latticed design of right hand. d) Abnormally low occipital hairline. e) Acanthosis nigricans of axillae. f) Small areas of incomplete alopecia. g) Cheilitis scrotalis. h) Scrotal tongue. i) Claw-like foot with wide space between big and second toes.

99

Pterygium syndrome (Status Bonnevie-Ullrich)

Pterygium colli is the main feature of the Bonnevie-Ullrich syndrome. Additional stigmata of this multifaceted disorder are congenital lymphangiectactic edema of the feet or neck, malformations of the extremities, dwarfism, pareses, hypoplasia of the muscles of the chest or abdominal wall, and an outward twisting of the elbows. The symmetry of these anomalies is noteworthy. Pterygium colli without evidence of Turner's syndrome occurs in familial cardiomyopathy (hypertrophy and fibrosis of the myocardium).

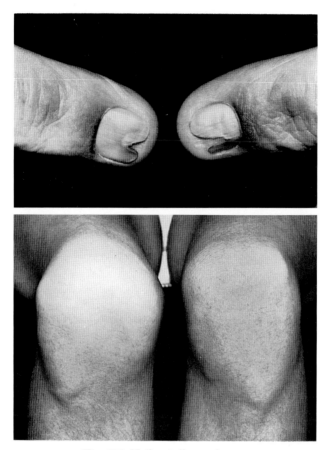

Fig. 172. Nail-patella syndrome

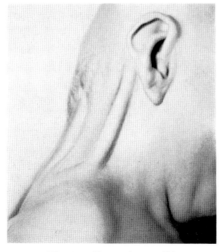

Fig. 174. Pterygium colli

12. Keratoses and Dystrophies

Diffuse keratoses (ichthyoses)

These anomalies of keratinization caused by abnormal genes are widely distributed over the body and may be classified into two main groups: 1. *Ichthyosis vulgaris* (with the subtypes of *Ichthyosis simplex, nitida, serpentina, nigricans, hystrix*, and *sauriasis*) characterized by noninvolvement of the flexor surfaces, aggravation in winter, and earliest manifestations around the first year of life, and 2. *Ichthyosis congenita* (with the subtypes *Ichthyosis congenita gravis* or *fetalis, mitis*, and *tarda* – congenital ichthyosiform erythroderma), characterized by involvement of the flexor surfaces, presence of manifestations at birth, and association with other anomalies.

Ichthyosis vulgaris

In ichthyosis vulgaris, lack of sweat and sebum, especially in winter, renders the integument dry, rough, or scaling. The conspicuous noninvolvement of the flexor surfaces and the axillae and the plate-like scales of the skin with desquamation in linear or quadrilateral figures are typical. *Ichthyosis localisata* represents an *ichthyosiform nevus*. The role of heredity in ichthyosis vulgaris is not fully understood (SCHNYDER). Dominant inheritance is unquestionably predominant; on the other hand, about 10 to 20 per cent of cases are inherited in an x-chromosomal recessive manner.

Ichthyosis congenita

The dirty-red, deeply fissured armour-plate skin of ichthyosis congenita is often particularly pronounced on the flexor surfaces. Other conspicuous stigmata are a flat nose (harlequin fetus), ectropion, abnormal configuration of ears, and sparse hair.

Collodion babies, children with "vernix caseosa persistens," are born in a slowly opening "cellophane" or "oil-paper" bag. Later – about the third or fourth month – they may exhibit symmetric spots on the knees. The fact that "fish-mouth" oral openings, eclabia, or rolled-in auricles are seen in this ichthyosis sebacea (HEBRA and KAPOSI), speaks in favor of the ano-

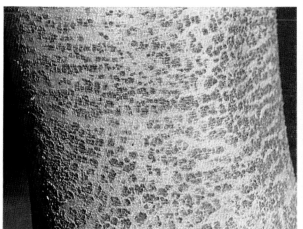

Fig. 175. Ichthyosis vulgaris (serpentina)

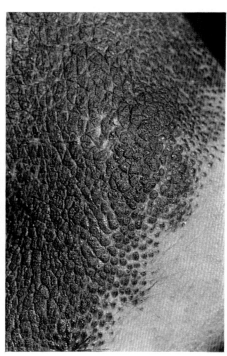

Fig. 176. Ichthyosiform nevus (localized ichthyosis)

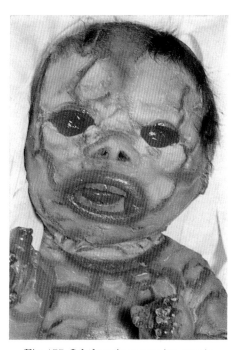

Fig. 177. Ichthyosis congenita gravis (Harlequin fetus)

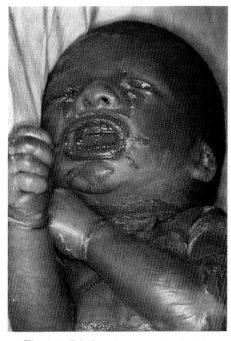

Fig. 178. Ichthyosis congenita fetalis

103

maly belonging to ichthyosis congenita mitis. Prognostically the disorder is predominantly favorable.

The dry form of congenital ichthyosiform erythroderma, inherited as a recessive trait and the bullous form, inherited as a dominant trait, are both "inflammatory"-exudative variants of ichthyosis congenita, which otherwise has to be considered a recessively inherited disorder (SCHNYDER). The history of the patient provides some clues for the diagnosis. Red skin at birth, increased growth of nails, and hunger for salt (BRUHNS) are characteristic.

Rud's syndrome (1927) is comprised of ichthyosis congenita, epilepsy, oligophrenia, hypogenitalism, partial gigantism, and polyneuritis; the *Sjögren-Larsson syndrome* (1957) refers to a related syndrome of ichthyosis congenita, spastic diplegia, in some instances retinal degeneration, disturbances of growth, and pernicious-like anemia.

The *Refsum syndrome* (1946) represents heredo-ataxia of cerebellar origin, associated with atypical retinitis pigmentosa, pupillary anomalies, polyneuritis, muscular atrophy, and ichthyosis (vulgaris), and has a varied, sometimes rather mild expression. The disorder may begin in adolescence or adulthood.

The enzyme defect of the Refsum syndrome occurs in the first stage of the alpha-oxidation of phytanic acid catabolism. It therefore belongs to the group of lipid storage diseases.

As LAUBENTHAL pointed out, *atypical ichthyosis* often accompanies various disturbances of the central nervous system.

Palmoplantar keratoses

Children show a lesser tendency toward keratinization than adults, and the usual trigger factors (such as mechanical exposure, arsenic, and trophoneuroses) do not yet play a role in the process. Thus, in this age group we rarely observe any symptomatic keratoses, but only small idiopathic palmoplantar keratoses (keratomas, keratodermas). Up to now about thirty phenotypes (with associated manifestations) are known. They are classified into three main forms.

Keratosis palmoplantaris diffusa (Thost, 1880; Unna, 1883)

This "perfect example of regular autosomal dominance" (SCHNYDER) rarely begins later than the first few weeks of life. The disorder assumes its full expression (marginal erythema, hyperhidrosis, sharply limited, diffuse, whitish-yellow hyperkeratoses with deep and painful rhagades) only after increasing mechanical pressure.

Special types: In *mal de Meleda* the hyperkeratoses progress beyond the palmar and plantar surfaces. The disorder begins in the first weeks of life. Its mode of inheritance may be recessive or dominant (GREITHER). In 1924 PAPILLON and LEFÈVRE described a strongly hyperhidrotic, transgressing *palmoplantar keratosis* with *periodontopathia* which gradually leads to complete loss of the teeth. *Keratosis palmoplantaris mutilans* (PARDO-COSTELLO and MESTRE; VOHWINKEL, 1929) also seems to be an hereditary disorder, which leads to constrictions that produce spontaneous ainhum-like amputations of fingers and toes, so-called dactylolysis spontanea.

Keratosis palmoplantaris insuliformis or striata

This rare, less hyperhidrotic type, described by Siemens, does not begin in the first weeks of life but late in childhood. Multiple other signs are frequently associated with the keratosis (keratosis multiformis).

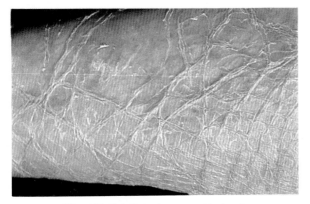

Fig. 180. Ichthyosis congenita tarda

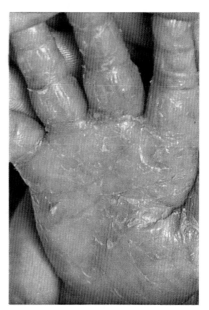

Fig. 179. Ichthyosis congenita fetalis.
Involvement of the hand

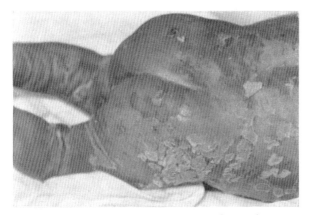

Fig. 181. Ichthyosis sebacea (collodion baby)

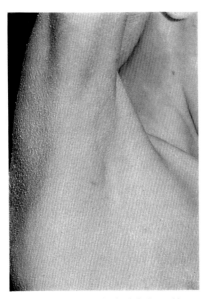

Fig. 182. Congenital ichthyosiform
erythroderma

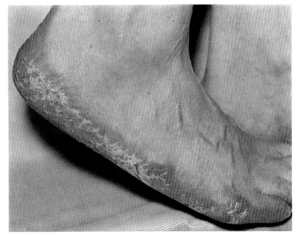

Fig. 183. Keratosis palmaris et plantaris hereditaria
diffusa (erythematous margin!)

105

Keratosis palmoplantaris papulosa (Buschke and Fischer, 1906; Brauer, 1913)

Regular autosomal dominant inheritance most probably governs this palmoplantar keratosis in which multiple small lesions are seen. Initially, pinhead to small pea-sized horny pearls are present. These fall off, leaving crater- or dimple-like depressions. These disseminated keratoses appear around the second or third decade, rarely in childhood.

Follicular keratoses

Keratosis follicularis lichenoides or lichen pilaris (T. Fox, 1875; Wilson, 1876)

This hyperkeratosis of the follicular orifices is most probably transmitted as an autosomal dominant characteristic. Manifestations are located predominantly on the extensor surfaces of the extremities. They occur around puberty, slightly more often in males. In women they regress around the climacteric. They create a crater-like aspect. The individual horny cones are either whitish or reddish and often terminate (particularly on the face) with atrophy (kératose pilaire rouge atrophiante de la face).

Another variety of keratosis pilaris rubra, having a different location (in the region of the eyebrows), occurs especially in blond individuals and begins in childhood. Ulerythema ophryogenes (TAENZER, 1889) is apparently a genodermatosis with an irregular dominant mode of inheritance. Characteristic is a thin, bandlike erythema with follicular keratosis. Later, there is a tendency to follicular atropy.

Semblances of these inherited follicular keratoses are engendered by lack of vitamin A (NICHOLLS: phrynoderma), vitamin C, or both. In the latter avitaminosis, a characteristic hemorrhagic component (e. g., lichen scorbuticus FESSNER), appears later in areas of goose pimples or crater-like follicular keratoses.

Keratosis follicularis spinulosa (Unna, Salinier)

These discontinuous, grouped, spinulous keratoses are associated with secondary pathologic reactions such as lichen scrofulosorum or trichophyticus, or with "spinulosism" in mycosis fungoides or follicular mucinosis in adults. The most important genodermatosis among the spinulous keratoses, present as early as the first weeks of life, is keratosis follicularis spinulosa decalvans (SIEMENS, 1925), which seems to be inherited as a dominant and sex-linked characteristic. The expression in heterozygous women is mild.

Keratosis follicularis acneiformis

These rather heterogeneous disorders are characterized by inflammatory comedo-like keratotic papules. They develop secondarily (occupational acne), affecting mainly adolescents exposed to certain occupational hazards.

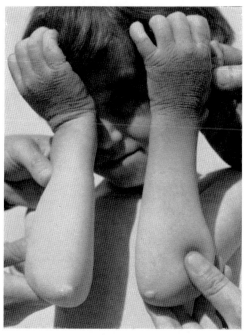

Fig. 184. Keratosis palmaris et plantaris diffusa
transgrediens (Mal de Meleda)

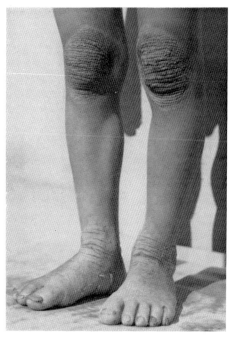

Fig. 185. Keratosis palmaris et plantaris
diffusa transgrediens (Mal de Meleda)

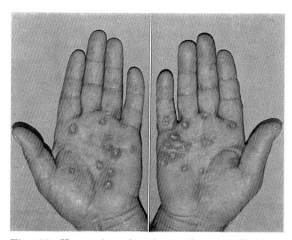

Fig. 186. Keratosis palmaris et plantaris dissipata

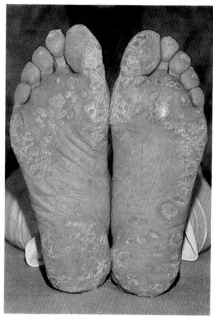

Fig. 187. Keratosis palmaris et plantaris
dissipata

Porokeratosis Mibelli (1893)

Keratoatrophic changes of hard, sharply demarcated, arciform, annular or striated horny ridges occur in both familial and isolated cases. The ridges consist of small, conical, horny excrescences which may fall off, leaving crater-like depressions. The extremities, the face, and the genitals are common sites. The disorder occurs most frequently in males.

Elastosis perforans serpiginosa

This dermatosis was originally described by LUTZ as *keratosis follicularis serpiginosa* and by MIESCHER as *elastoma intrapapillare perforans* because of dystrophic alterations of the elastic tissue. Occurring chiefly in adolescents, it is found in the neck region in the form of closely aggregated, verrucous papules in annular or serpiginous distribution. Apparently, other congenital anomalies (cutis laxa, osteogenesis imperfecta, congenital poikilodermas, and so forth) may be associated.

Keratosis follicularis et parafollicularis in cutem penetrans (KYRLE, 1916) does not present in annular distribution but rather in isolated, distinctly elevated, verrucous, horny thickenings; it also differs pathohistologically from elastosis perforans serpiginosa.

Dyskeratosis follicularis (Darier)

In 1889 DARIER, jointly with THIBAUT, erroneously described this genodermatosis as an infectious disorder (psorospermosis). The dermatosis often occurs sporadically. Its earliest manifestations are seen in the first or second decade, or even in early infancy. It has a tendency to grouping and to foul-smelling vegetations which may be found on sites in which seborrhea is likely to occur, that is, the intertriginous areas. The single lesion is reddish or grayish-red, fatty, easily crumbled, squamous or crusted, and located at or near the site of the follicle*. If the fully developed horny cone is lifted up, the thumb-nail shape of the horny lamella is easily recognized. On the dorsa of the hands large, flat, wartlike papular lesions predominate. On the lower back, however, white spots are frequently observed, and these may represent initial changes. The mucous membranes are almost always affected. The nails show longitudinal grooves, striated discolorations, and disintegration, corresponding to the dyskeratoses on the rest of the skin. Even more characteristic are the interruptions of the papillary ridges of the fingerprints. Lesions are provoked by light, and the condition usually worsens during the summer.

Acanthosis nigricans (Pollitzer and Janovsky, 1890)

This pigmentary, papillary dystrophy is accompanied by itching. The intertriginous areas (genitoanal, axillary, and submammary) are sites of predilection. Malignant acanthosis nigricans appears after the fortieth year** and is associated with adenocarcinoma of the gastrointestinal tract, ovary, breast, lung, and so forth.

---

* In spite of the name keratosis follicularis, the site of the process is not limited to the follicle. *The translators.*

** Any case of acanthosis nigricans after puberty in a nonobese individual suggests the malignant type. Children only rarely suffer from this type. *The translators.*

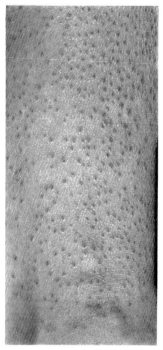

Fig. 188. Keratosis follicularis
lichenoides (lichen pilaris)

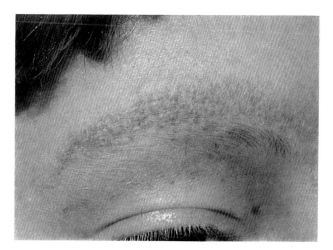

Fig. 189. Ulerythema ophryogenes

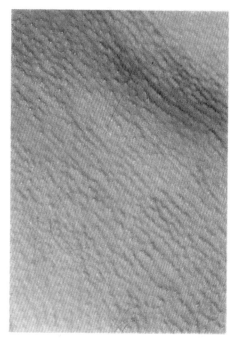

Fig. 190. Keratosis follicularis spinulosa

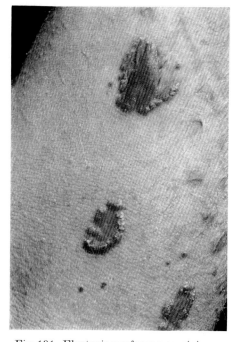

Fig. 191. Elastosis perforans serpiginosa

Distinct from this malignant type is pseudoacanthosis nigricans (OLLENDORFF CURTH), which occurs in obese dark-complexioned individuals of any age. Children may be affected. (The obesity may be caused by endocrine disturbances, among other factors. *The translators.*) More discrete lesions appearing in the same locations are known as confluent and reticulated papillomatosis. Occasionally, small associated pedunculated fibromas may be found. *Benign* acanthosis nigricans is present at birth or begins in childhood or at puberty. It resembles ichthyosis hystrix and is not accompanied by endocrine disturbances. It is transmitted in an irregularly dominant fashion. *The translators.*

Pseudoxanthoma elasticum

Pseudoxanthoma elasticum was described by RIGAL in 1881, by BALZER in 1881, and by CHAUFFARD in 1889. DARIER, however, in 1896 described the histopathology of Chauffard's case and gave the disorder its name. The disorder represents a systemic, metabolic, dysplastic elastosis rather than a degenerative process. Apparently, recessive inheritance is observed more often than dominant inheritance (WISE). The cardinal signs usually appear in the first or second decade but in rare instances may be present at birth. The ivory-white to lemon-yellow striated reticular, papular or macular lesions sometimes show thin telangiectases. The lesions are located on the sides of the neck, the axillae, the folds of the large joints, and occasionally on the inner aspects of the thighs and the genitocrural folds. The ocular fundus shows brownish-yellow streaks of branching blood vessels ("angioid streaks"), which were first described in 1929 by the ophthalmologist E. GRÖNBLAD and the dermatologist STRANDBERG. This phenomenon is also observed in about 10 per cent of patients with Paget's disease. In addition, there are cardiovascular signs (angina pectoris!) and vascular changes of the medium-sized and smaller arteries (for example, asymptomatic blocking of the ulnar and radial arteries, and intermittent claudication.) Changes similar to those observed on the skin are found in the gastrointestinal tract (oral cavity, stomach, and rectum). An important additional phenomenon of the systemic elastorrhexis is the tendency to calcification, which may also have a genetic basis.

110

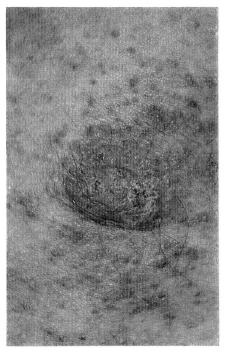

Fig. 192. Darier's disease
(disseminated papules on areas exposed
to light)

Fig. 193. Darier's disease
(confluent and closely disseminated
papules)

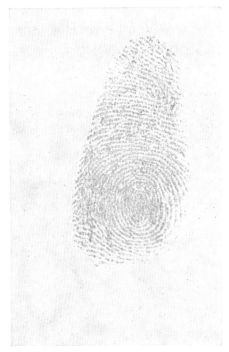

Fig. 194. Darier's disease
(characteristic interruptions of the
dermatoglyphics)

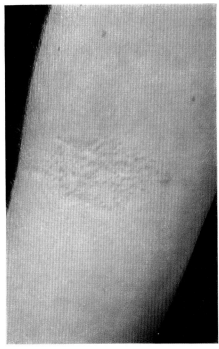

Fig. 195. Pseudoxanthoma elasticum

13. Bullous Dermatoses

Pemphigus

Here we will discuss 1. the pemphigus group with *acanthoytic blister formation*, pemphigus congenitus (epidermolysis hereditaria), and 2. the most important specific *skin reactions with subepidermal blister formation*, chiefly, *dermatitis herpetiformis*.

Acute malignant pemphigus of the last century represents, as discussed before, the same disease as the Lyell syndrome and therefore corresponds in infants to dermatitis exfoliativa neonatorum (V. RITTERSHAIN).

It must be admitted that chronic pemphigus, the bullous disease, hardly ever occurs in children; such a diagnosis should therefore be made only with the greatest care. Of the three forms of chronic pemphigus, only *pemphigus vulgaris* (WICHMANN, 1791) occurs in children. Instances of pemphigus between the fourth and the fifteenth years of life comprise only 5 per cent of all cases of pemphigus.

In contrast, *pemphigus foliaceus* (CAZENAVE, 1844), a variety also starting with bullae, but soon changing to a laminated pastry-like, squamo-crusted erythroderma, comprises only 1 per cent of all cases of pemphigus in children. *Pemphigus vegetans* (I. NEUMANN, 1896) is believed to show the same incidence.

A characteristic diagnostic sign of *chronic pemphigus*, especially of the vulgaris variety, is the arbitrary development (with regard to time and location) of unilocular, first taut, then collapsing, and later turbid bullae on normal skin (criterion of NODET), a process which most probably arises from a loosening of tonofibrils on an autoimmune basis. This seems to be proved by fluorescence of the serum, which shows fixation of the antibodies in the serum to the intercellular substance of the squamous cell epithelium. As a consequence of the acantholysis (AUSPITZ, 1881; CIVATTE, 1943) the bullous cover or the normal-appearing skin surrounding it can, on tangential pressure, be easily moved (NIKOLSKY's phenomenon). The intraepidermal site of the bulla permits healing without residua. At most, the skin shows pigmentation. On the mucous membranes, there are often only preliminary blisters present, that is, yellowish-white epithelial membranes, shiny, moist lesions, and open erosions.

Senear-Usher syndrome

The facial lesions in *pemphigus erythematosus* simulate lupus erythematosus; lesions on other parts of the body look like seborrheic eczema and pemphigus foliaceus.

113

Dermatitis herpetiformis (Duhring, 1884)

This highly polymorphous ("wide-spectrum") dermatosis exhibits periodic activity. The general well-being of the afflicted individual is not impaired, except for sensations of severe pruritus or a peculiar painful burning sensation. The eruption has a conspicuous symmetry, shows a tendency to grouping, and favors the posterior axillary fold. It consists of erythemas, wheals, blisters (in preponderantly herpetiform distribution), bullae, a few pustules, and occasionally monosymptomatic prurigo eruptions with their characteristic sequence of secondary lesions (scales, crusts, and so forth). Additional features are the tendency to eosinophilia in the hemogram and the contents of the blisters, and an idiosyncrasy to halogens, particularly iodine (iodized table salt or salt water fish). This idiosyncrasy has been used as a diagnostic test, either epicutaneously (with 30 per cent potassium iodide in vaseline), or, more often, orally (with a few drops of Lugol's solution in a glass of water). Dermatitis herpetiformis, however, represents a disorder with many causes, so that every instance of the disease needs thorough investigation for food allergy, infestation with worms, bacterial infections, visceral neoplasms, or other causes.

In children, in contrast to adults, favored locations are the face, genitals, buttocks, and lower abdomen. Moreover, up to the third year of life children show fewer papulovesicular lesions and many more bullous lesions (so-called pemphigus juvenilis). There also may be a stage of grouped prurigo-lesions on the knees and elbows in adolescents. Whereas in adults it is common to see the first attack quickly becoming superinfected and accompanied by fever and lymphadenopathy, the course of recurrent attacks in children is more protracted and less violent. Puberty often marks the end of the disorder.

Bullous pemphigoid

This chronic disorder of limited duration was differentiated from pemphigus by LEVER in 1953 (PRAKKEN and WOERDEMANN named it parapemphigus). It occurs infrequently in children but frequently in old people (*pemphigus of old age*, STEIGLEDER). The formation of blisters in these "bullous pemphigoids" takes place in the subepidermal zone of the corium. Not only this fact, but also the almost exclusive presence of multiple large blisters, speak in favor of this disorder belonging at least macroscopically to the exquisitely bullous variety of dermatitis herpetiformis. Histologically, however, important considerations (such as absence of peribullous abscesses) favor a separation of bullous pemphigoid from dermatitis herpetiformis.

Benign mucous membrane pemphigoid (essential shrinkage of the mucous membranes)

This name denotes the attempt to give another name to "pemphigus conjunctivae". Its so-called benign character is not discernible with the frequent development of fibrous adhesions, scars, conjunctival adhesions, and esophageal strictures. In the French literature ocular pemphigus is also called "dermatite bulleuse muco-synéchiante et atrophiante de LORTAT-JACOB."

Subcorneal pustular dermatosis (Sneddon and Wilkinson, 1956)

This dermatosis, either related to or even identical with dermatitis herpetiformis, affects women over the age of 20 almost exclusively. The distinctive feature is the croplike appearance

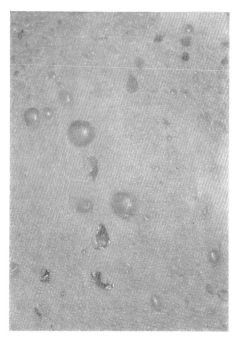

Fig. 196. Chronic pemphigus vulgaris
(bullae on skin)

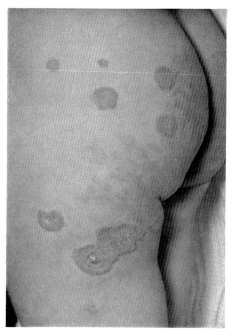

Fig. 197. Dermatitis herpetiformis Duhring.
(Gyrate urticarial erythematous lesions)

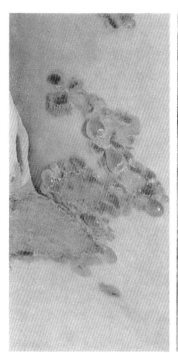

Fig. 198. Dermatitis herpetiformis Duhring. (Peripheral
bullae on an erythematous base)

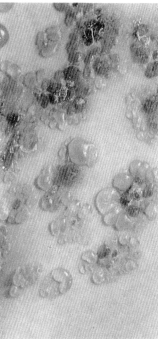

Fig. 199. Dermatitis herpetiformis Duhring. (Vesicles in
herpetiform distribution)

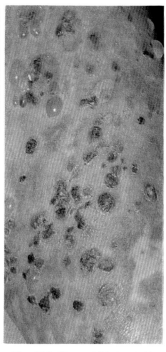

Fig. 200. Dermatitis herpetiformis Duhring.
(Characteristic polymorphism)

115

of groups of vesicles and pustules which have a tendency to form thin, arciform, crusted and scaling single figures. In children, one should keep the diagnosis of *impetigo circinata* in mind.

Familial benign chronic pemphigus (Hailey and Hailey)

This disease affects children infrequently. As a rule, persons over 30 years manifest grouped blisters on limited areas (neck, nape, axillae, and genitocrural folds). These are transformed into circinate, moderately vegetating, spongy, grayish-red lesions. Inheritance is that of irregular dominance.

Bullous genodermatoses (epidermolysis group)

This whole group, in which there is a considerable variety of manifestations, is based on a genetically conditioned structural weakness in the area of the basal layer and adjacent layers. Clinically, this defect presents "an hereditary tendency to blister formation" (GOLD-SCHEIDER, 1892), called "epidermolysis bullosa hereditaria" (KÖBNER, 1896). Essentially, this is a "bullosis *mechanica* hereditaria" (SIEMENS), since the blister formation, noticeable as early as in infancy but definitely evident with the first attempts at walking, is dependent on slight mechanical stress. Less conspicuous is the dependency on warm weather or warm baths, as observed chiefly by COCKAYNE (1938), who named the disorder "recurrent blister-ous eruption of the feet in hot weather." From this tardive minimal variation which frequently affects only the palms and soles to the fully developed picture of epidermolysis bullosa hereditaria, all grades of involvement are observed.

Epidermolysis bullosa hereditaria simplex

This disorder is inherited in an autosomal dominant mode. It distinctly favors the male sex. In contrast to other types, changes of the nails and mucous membranes are usually absent. At different ages a certain similarity to pemphigus syphiliticus, dermatitis exfoliativa von Rittershain, acrodermatitis enteropathica, or a form of porphyria is evident.

Epidermolysis bullosa hereditaria dystrophica dominans

Here, the subepidermal site of the blisters and certain changes in the elastic tissue cause characteristic scarring, atrophy, or keloid formation, and, above all, postbullous horny cysts (milia). In this dystrophic form of epidermolysis (COCKAYNE-TOURAINE) the oral and conjunctival mucous membranes may also be affected. Additional features are claw-like sclerodactylia, dystrophic nails, and palmoplantar hyperhidrosis.

PASINI's (1926) dominant dystrophic epidermolysis bullosa albopapuloidea is probably a separate genetic entity, affecting the extremities, the trunk, and the lumbosacral area. It shows cobble stone-like or fat, torpid, elevated, ivory-colored plaques. The few lesions or multiple small patches present usually develop in the second decade.

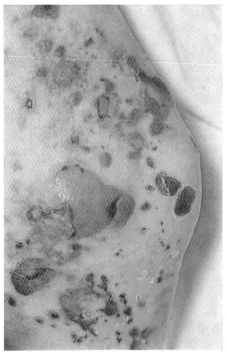

Fig. 201. Bullous pemphigoid

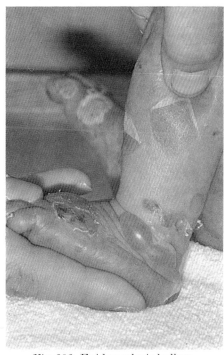

Fig. 202. Epidermolysis bullosa
hereditaria (Nikolski sign)

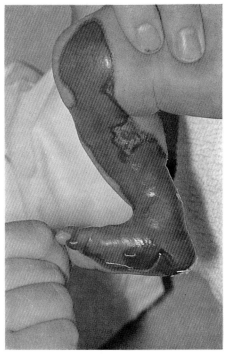

Fig. 203. Epidermolysis bullosa
hereditaria

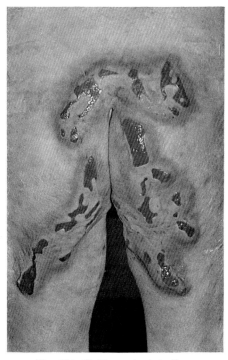

Fig. 204. Epidermolysis bullosa
hereditaria hyperplastica

Epidermolysis bullosa hereditaria dystrophica recessiva (Hallopeau-Siemens)

The main features of this recessive dystrophic variety, often called *epidermolysis bullosa hereditaria dystrophica polydysplastica* (TOURAINE), are rather early or late severe involvement of the mucous membranes as far down as the esophagus (stenosis), dystrophic nails, and anomalies of the hair and teeth. Severe forms show impairment of skeletal function and mutilations.

Pediatricians have considered *epidermolysis bullosa letalis* (HERLITZ, 1935) as probably a new entity. Blisters on skin and mucous membranes heal without sequelae, but onychodystrophy and skeletal atrophies are present. This is a disorder of autosomal recessive inheritance, showing greater familial involvement and a grave prognosis for life.

14. Cutaneous Reactions to Physical and Chemical Agents

Three stages are recognized in thermal burns, scalds, and frostbite: first degree, erythema; second degree, blister formation; and third degree, necrosis. Evaluation of the extent and depth of the damage and its prognosis can be determined correctly only after hours, and sometimes days. Generally speaking, the outlook is more serious in children. Some authors recommend expressing the extent of the cutaneous damage in terms of per cent of the total body surface and multiplying it by three in children between the ages of 1 and 4 years and by two in children between the ages of 4 to 12. Whereas in adults involvement of half to two-thirds of the surface renders the prognosis hopeless, in children involvement of a smaller area is grave. In contrast to the dramatic course of a severe burn, with its anhydremia, hypoproteinemia, drop in colloid osmotic pressure, increase in potassium, and disturbances of microcirculation, the general reaction to *congelation* is much less evident. Later, a toxemic phase develops for which (according to modern concepts) endogenous toxins (including histamine) are less responsible than the liberated proteases of the tissue, and, most important, the bacterial toxins.

As far as secondary infection of burns is concerned, one should always consider the possibility of tetanus. The threat of scarlet fever arising at the site of burned skin exists in young children. This type of scarlet fever exanthem does not differ from scarlatiniform eruptions of different origin. It may be accompanied by sore throat, raspberry tongue, and so forth. Scarlet fever may develop within hours of, but also one to two weeks after, the burn. Burns may lead to gastric or intestinal ulcers, and for this reason the amount of corticosteroids that can be given to mitigate shock or toxemia is limited. A frequent aftereffect of burns is the development of characteristic keloids.

Frostbite begins at the acra in a definitely symmetric distribution; chiefly toes, fingers, ears, and nose are damaged. The clinical picture itself, with distinct individual differences, is complete only after a certain time interval. W. SCHNEIDER sees the reason for this delay in the damaging effect of cold on the more deeply located sensitive blood vessels; heat damages the more superficial cutaneous layers.

Implantation of foreign bodies is seen in infants. When objects are imbedded in previously existing wounds they are subsequently enclosed in the scar (tattooing); in later life this is frequently an occupational hazard. It is well known that cutaneous implantation of a piece of indelible ink pencil is hardly painful, but it may cause tissue necrosis complicated by lymphangitis. Spines of cacti and similar plants may lead to abscesses and felons, especially on the hands and fingers. Occasionally they may later lead to tuberculoid or sarcoidal granulomas.

Alkaline substances produce colliquative necroses, whereas acids cause sharply outlined coagulative necroses. Too often, children develop deep cauterizations when crystalline agents (such as silver nitrate and potassium permanganate) added to water for irrigations or baths have not been sufficiently dissolved and contact the skin in concentrated form.

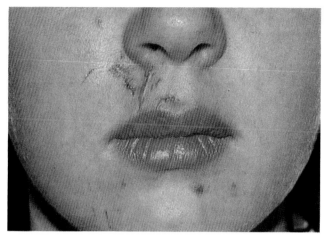
Fig. 205. Tattoo marks caused by dirt

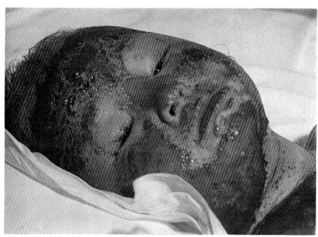
Fig. 206. Second degree burn

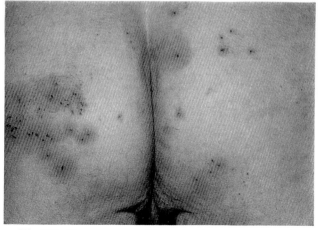
Fig. 207. Necroses caused by potassium permanganate
crystals (in sitz bath)

15. Photodermatoses

Xeroderma pigmentosum

The porphyrias and related disorders are discussed under metabolic disorders. Xeroderma pigmentosum (KAPOSI, 1870) is hardly compatible with a normal life. This photodermatosis is usually inherited as an autosomal recessive trait, rarely as an autosomal dominant trait. It manifests itself in the early years of life when the individual with this disposition is exposed to sunlight. The hypersensitivity to the rays of the sun is genetically transmitted, but deficient adaptation to light is also evident (an important feature is the fast-appearing and long-maintained hyperpigmentation following doses of alpine light). If exposure to light continues, diffuse melanoderma ensues and genetically determined abnormal pigmented nevi, partly like ephelides, partly like lentigines, appear (POPOFF: ephelidosis maligna). These are later associated with atrophic poikilodermatous changes. Finally, there are mutilations, with a preference for the auricles, nose, and lids (entropion or others). As an expression of premature skin senility, verrucous keratoses develop, on the basis of which squamous cell and basal cell carcinomas, sarcomas, and rarely even melanomas may appear. LANGHOF found in such cases increased copper and lowered glutathione values in the serum, and amino acids in the urine.

Solar urticaria

This is a rare form of physical allergy. Different types are determined by the wavelengths of the light source. Most patients respond to rays below the wavelength of 3700 Å.

Familial protoporphyrinemic solar urticaria (LANGHOF, MUELLER, and RIETSCHE) is discussed with the porphyrias.

Solar dermatitis and chronic polymorphic light eruptions

Hydroa aestivale and *hydroa vacciniformis* (BAZIN) are at present classified as being related to the congenital porphyrias. Proof, however, is hardly available. *Solar dermatitis*, with a tendency to lichenification of the exposed parts of the body, and *chronic polymorphic* (erythematous, erthematoid, pruriginous) *light eruptions* are seen primarily in girls or women, in the early sunny season. Later, diminished hypersensitivity to light follows, even with increased sunlight. A spontaneous remission with decreased exposure to sunlight,

122

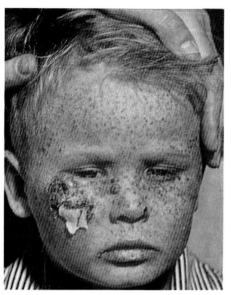

Fig. 208. Xeroderma pigmentosum

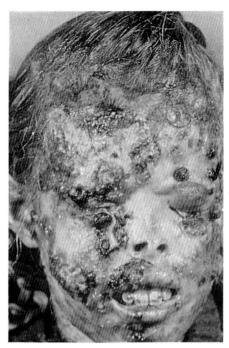

Fig. 209. Xeroderma pigmentosum

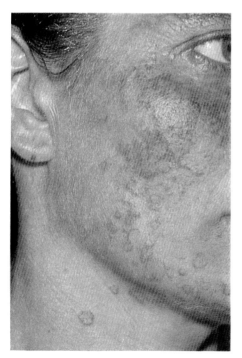

Fig. 210. Polymorphic light eruption

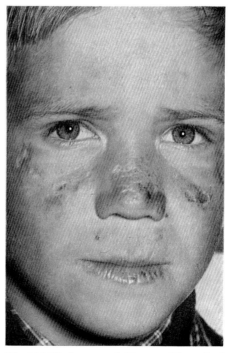

Fig. 211. Hydroa vacciniforme with marked
scar formation

however, may be observed. According to WISKEMAN and WULF an especially harmful effect is exerted chiefly by longwave ultraviolet light, ranging from 320 to 400 Å. The presence of protein derivatives of tryptophane metabolism (KIMMIG: light-band products or indolyl-acryloglycine) in the urine are of diagnostic value.

Perniosis of spring

In 1940 KEINING named this photodermatosis *perniosis of spring*. In 1942 BUCKHARDT called it *solar dermatosis of spring*. Primarily children are affected. They present papulo-vesicular eruptions, mostly on the rims of the ears but also on the dorsa of the fingers. The lesions recur every year and regress spontaneously.

Phototoxic and photoallergic reactions

Phototoxic reactions are those with direct absorption of rays by light-absorbing substances; photoallergic reactions, the knowledge of which we owe to EPSTEIN and BURKHARDT, are those eruptions caused by light in addition to the photosensitizing substances (TRONNIER). Photosensitivity, which follows in every case and is not an allergic phenomenon in the usual sense of the word, frequently occurs as *phytophotodermatosis*, such as *dermatitis bullosa striata pratensis* (OPPENHEIM and FESSLER), *grass dermatitis*, or *berloque dermatitis* (FREUND-ROSENTHAL) which, as well as *photodermatitis pigmentata* (IPPEN), is caused by oil of bergamot, i. e., furocumarin (KUSKE). Photoallergies (to sulfonamides, including oral anti-diabetic drugs, hydrochlorothiazides, phenothiazides, some antifungal drugs, and others) usually occur in adults. In children demethyltetracycline, known also because of its ability to discolor teeth, can lead to *photoonycholysis*.

A common example of a *phototraumatic reaction* following an overdose of shortwave ultra-violet light is acute sunburn, *acute solar dermatitis*. It begins with a macular, follicular, later confluent erythema, occasionally with formation of bullae, and is sometimes accompanied by vomiting, syncope, and other complications.

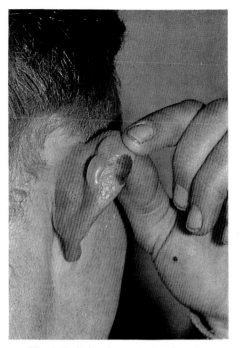

Fig. 212. Solar dermatosis of spring

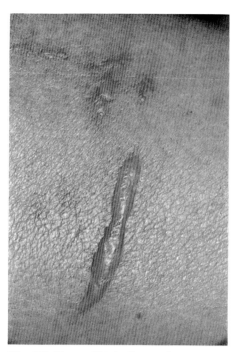

Fig. 213. Dermatitis bullosa striata pratensis (dermatitis due to plants growing in a
meadow)

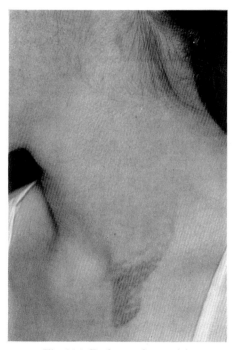

Fig. 214. Berloque dermatitis

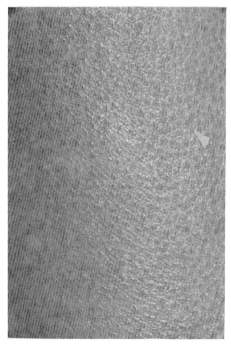

Fig. 215. Acute solar dermatitis (sunburn)
beginning with follicular erythema

16. Pigmentary Disturbances

The process of melanogenesis is complex. The central regulation of pigment is influenced in a positive way by melanocyte-stimulating hormones, synthesized in the median lobe of the hypophysis; melatonin (LERNER), on the other hand, is supposed to offset this mechanism, at least in amphibious skin. Melatonin is synthesized in man in the pineal body and, being chemically a substitute for serotonin, is related to tryptophane metabolism. Ultraviolet light can directly (by oxidation of chromogenes weak in color) or indirectly (through an erythema caused by exposure to light) lead to tanning of the skin. Clinically noticeable in children is the increase in melanin after regression of even the most banal dermatoses, such as scabies, infestation with lice, or staphylogenous impetigo. In contrast is post-lesional depigmentation, such as leukoderma after secondary syphilis, psoriasis vulgaris, parapsoriasis guttata, pityriasis rosea, and rarely after chickenpox.

Melanodermas

The first group of congenital hyperpigmentations are the acropigmentations, reported in detail chiefly by Japanese authors. *Acropigmentation* was also described by Thomas in 1923. This rather frequently observed and almost physiologic picture of melanin hyperpigmentation occurs around the fingernails and toenails of children. It slowly regresses around the fifth or sixth year. Just as common are *ephelides* (freckles). Their development is determined by genetic as well as environmental factors. Pigmented nevi (local accumulations of melanin without nevus formations), such as *nevi spili* and *lentigines*, which occur as part of syndromes, will be discussed with the phakomatoses. Hyperpigmentations caused by hormonal disturbances and influenced by active and mechanical factors occur in childhood almost solely in Addison's disease and in (incomplete) addisonism. Yellow to bronze coloring is found, predominantly in the lines of the hand, on the nipples, in the genitoanal area, but it may also occur as spots on the oral mucosa. The gums present pigmentation comparable to the line resulting from lead poisoning. Of the numerous types of chloasma (uterinum, "biliary mask," brown ring on forehead*), adolescents manifest chiefly the circumoral pigmentary erythrosis of BROCQ, in which there is pigmentation as well as a faint telangiectatic erythema.

---

* Lately, chloasma has been observed in women taking contraceptive pills. *The translators.*

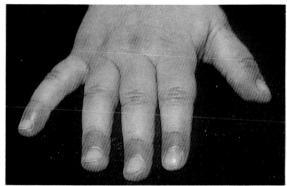

Fig. 216. Acropigmentation

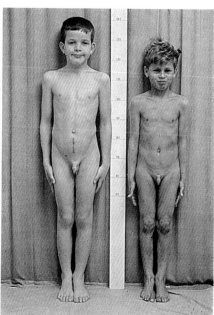

Fig. 217. Addison's disease (child on the right)

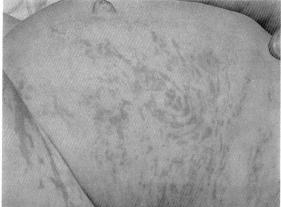

Fig. 218. Incontinentia pigmenti

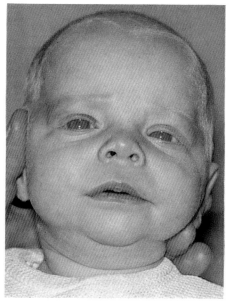

Fig. 220. Albinism

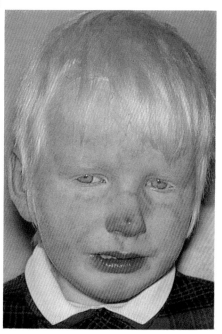

Fig. 219. Albinism

A unique pigmentary dermatosis in childhood is incontinentia pigmenti (BLOCH-SULZBER-GER), which occurs predominantly in girls. Its initial lesions are present at birth or in the first months of life. The dermatosis represents a pigmentary anomaly with characteristic configurations branching out like deer antlers, or spattered, open or reticular, slate-gray or fudge-like pigmentation. At an early stage it is also associated with high eosinophilia of the blood and tissues and shows pinhead to lentil-sized inflammatory (urticarial) papulo-pustular or lineally arranged bullous lesions, which appear in crops. The whole picture, then, is reminiscent of Duhring's disease. The general well-being of the patient is rarely impaired. In contrast to dermatitis herpetiformis, however, the inflammatory lesions of incontinentia pigmenti are gone after one year, at the latest. But before characteristic pigmentations develop there may be a new shower of again lineally arranged lichenoid, hyperkeratotic, or verrucoid lesions. In addition, there are cerebral (convulsions), ophthalmologic (glioma, cataract), osseous, and cardiac (congenital cardiac defects) manifestations and disturbances of dentition.

Most of the 100 cases observed suggested a genetically based disorder. In a few cases, however, the history points to an embryopathia caused by a viral infection during pregnancy (UEBEL, LUDWIG, and KORTING). Infrequently, there are disturbances of the growth of nails and the hair. If the pigmentary changes do not branch out but are instead reticular, we are dealing with a pigmentary dermatosis belonging to the type of "familial chromatophore nevus" of NAEGELI.

Leukopathias

The cause of genetically determined albinism is not the congenital absence or diminution of melanin in skin, hair, and the pigment-bearing ocular membranes; origin of the disorder lies chiefly in the blockage of the enzyme tyrosinase in the melanocytes, which themselves are not impaired (FITZPATRICK and LERNER). Albinism exists in complete or incomplete (albinoidism) forms; it also exists in a localized form, for example, the white forelock (poliosis circumscripta). Outstanding in complete albinism is the conspicuous ocular involvement, characterized by a red iris and horizontal nystagmus. The inheritance of ocular albinism (albinism solum bulbi, solum fundi) is sex-linked. A special type is the syndrome of KLEIN and WAARDENBURG, which shows localized albinism, deaf-mutism, blepharophimosis, dystopia of the lower openings of the lacrimal ducts, and hypoplasia of the iris. Another special type of localized albinism or nevus depigmentosus is Sutton's nevus or leukoderma acquisitum centrifugum. In both forms, as a single spot or multiple lesions, it represents either the combination of a nevus cell nevus (less frequently of a different nevus) with a nevus depigmentosus, or represents vitiligo in perinevoid distribution. The absence of peripheral hyperpigmentation of the white halo speaks against this concept. Typical vitiligo usually shows such hyperpigmentation.

Vitiligo is an acquired, idiopathic (primary, without preexisting changes) leukopathia. The affected areas are sharply circumscribed. The dermatosis usually starts around the anogenital region. It is symmetrically distributed and the border of the affected areas is characterized by hyperpigmentation. Development of the dermatosis is slow. Its distribution does not show any relationship to the nerves or the blood vessels. The cause of vitiligo is considered by PINKUS to be a loss of function of tyrosinase of the melanocytes at the junction. LERNER, on the other hand, assumes that a melatonin-like substance is excreted at the peripheral

Fig. 221. Nevus depigmentosus

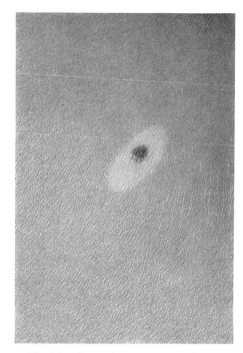

Fig. 222. Sutton's nevus (leukoderma acquisitum centrifugum)

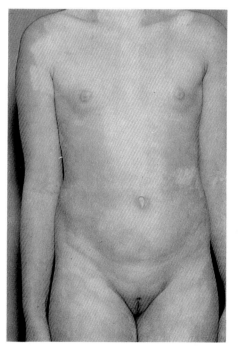

Fig. 223. Vitiligo

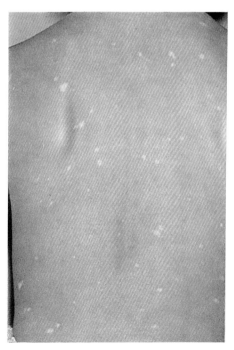

Fig. 224. Secondary depigmentation (leukoderma) following varicella

129

nerve endings of the skin, lightening the pigment cell and blocking neomelanogenesis. Dominant inheritance seems to be the mode of transmission. It seems that sporadic cases of vitiligo do not occur as often as has been assumed, because in about 20 to 30 per cent of observed cases familial involvement is noted. According to LERNER's extensive studies, in more than 50 per cent of patients vitiligo occurs before the twentieth year of life.

17. Circulatory and Vascular Disorders of the Skin

Common circulatory disorders

Organic circulatory disease in childhood or adolescence is hardly of any importance; however, angioneuropathies and angiopathies have been observed. Such terms describe pathologic conditions (of only negligible clinical importance) of the upper vascular plexus of the cutis with either vasodilatory or constricting reactivity.

Acrocyanosis (BROCQ) consists of a spastic-atonic syndrome (O. MÜLLER) with marked dilatation of the venules accompanied by severe vasoconstriction of the arterioles. During the lifetime of a patient with a labile vasomotoric system there is a distinct dependence on the endocrine system. As a rule the lesions regress between the ages of 20 and 25. They may recur, however, and become more severe at the preclimacteric period. In acrocyanosis, areas which have become anemic upon pressure with a finger return to normal concentrically, beginning at the periphery. (Parrisius's phenomenon of the "iris diaphragm of the microscope".) Cinnabar-red or circumscribed anemic areas interspersed with large patches of blue discoloration are typical. A clinical variant of acrocyanosis is *erythrocyanosis crurum puellarum* (KLINGMÜLLER) (bluish discoloration of the legs of young women), which, in contrast to the localized areas of frostbite, is widespread, with increased follicular markings (perniosis follicularis; KLINGMÜLLER; DITTRICH). Similar persistent vasomotoric erythemas occur on the cheeks and the nose and are constitutional. Such patients belong to the so-called "rustic type" (MONCORPS).

On the faces of children, essential telangiectases which resemble persistent erythemas may be the result of strangulation during labor. Frostbite results in circumscribed, bluish-red, frequently nodular swellings, chiefly on the hands, feet, and legs. The affected areas will characteristically start to itch as they become warmer. Endogenous constitutional factors again play a predisposing role for damage by cold.

Of the livedo conditions of the skin, the superficial blotchy type with a constant reticulated pattern and no subjective symptoms is *cutis marmorata*. The white negative picture of this condition is cutis marmorata alba (COMEL). The condition is caused by a deep local vascular hypertonia. *Congenital telangiectatic cutis marmorata* (LOHUIZEN) has already been mentioned as a nevoid malformation.

131

Cutis marmorata and *livedo reticularis* (KAPOSI) are to a large extent considered synonymous. *Ehrmann's livedo racemosa* shows the same lightning-like or reticulated bizarre configuration, but its underlying pathologic-anatomic basis is a vascular change of the walls (endoarteriolitis or endophlebitis). Formerly, livedo racemosa was thought to be almost exclusively a sign of syphilis or tuberculosis. Nowadays periarteritis nodosa and endangiitis obliterans are considered to be causative factors.

Periarteritis nodosa

The classic form of periarteritis (KUSSMAUL and MAIER, 1866) is rare in infants, children, or the aged. Cutaneous changes are to be expected in about 20 to 40 per cent of the cases. The changes present as hemorrhagic, nodular, or papulonecrotic lesions, which may progress to a condition called "apoplexia cutis" (F. FREUND). Livedo racemosa has been mentioned previously as a possible manifestation of periarteritis nodosa.

Arteriolitis "allergica" cutis

RUITER (1957) classified as such a group of clinical manifestations (maladie trisymptomatique de GOUGEROT, "allergides nodulaires dermiques," and similar conditions) which show similar pathologic changes of the small blood vessels, chiefly in the corium. These primary cutaneous vasculitides are characterized by inflammatory reactions and fibrinoid changes, and present a polymorphic clinical appearance with urticarial, hemorrhagic, papulonecrotic, or nodular lesions.

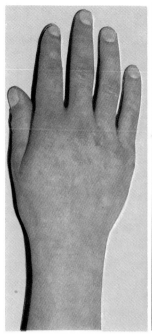

Fig. 225. Acrocyanosis
with Bier's spots

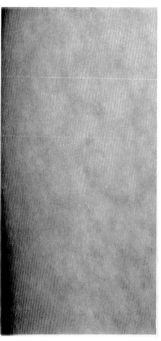

Fig. 226. Cutis marmorata

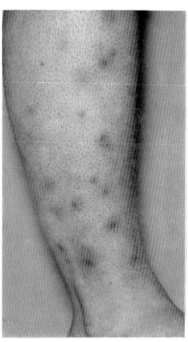

Fig. 229. Hyperergic arteriolitis

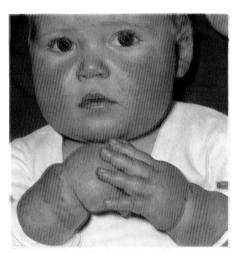

Fig. 227. Acute frostbite

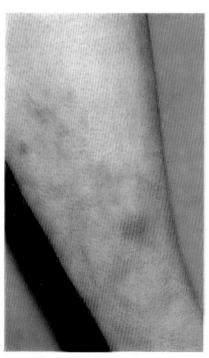

Fig. 228. Follicular frostbite

18. Hemorrhagic Diatheses

VIRCHOW (1854) developed this concept to describe conditions of abnormal bleeding from the various body openings or into the skin, mucous membranes, or internal organs. This includes disturbances of hemostasis which are dependent upon the following components: blood vessels, thrombocytes, and plasma (and their respective coagulation factors). Cutaneous and extracutaneous hemorrhagic lesions are classified – according to the frequency with which they are observed in dermatologic practice – as vascular, thrombocytic, and coagulation defects. Only the most frequently occurring special types of particular age groups will be mentioned.

Vascular disorders

Angiopathies (vascular disorders) which frequently develop only on small areas or as secondary hemorrhagic lesions are represented by punctate petechial lesions rather than by diffuse macular lesions (suffusions).

Hereditary hemorrhagic telangiectasia (Osler's disease)

Well known among the congenital vascular hemorrhagic diatheses is Rendu-Osler disease, characterized by episodes of bleeding from the nose, lungs, intestinal tract, or vagina, and cutaneous hemorrhages subungually or into the volar aspects of fingers or toes. The area of the midface shows either angiomas or spider nevi. Simple ampullary vascular dilatations or convolutions of dysplastic vessels with obstruction of arteries and arteriovenous anastomoses are present histologically; they are quantitatively and qualitatively influenced by various stimuli. The disease is inherited in autosomal dominant fashion. During the early phase with epistaxis, angiomas are prevalent. Later, angiectatic lesions, occasionally accompanied by cirrhosis of the liver, are more common.

Schönlein-Henoch purpura and Möller-Barlow disease

Möller-Barlow disease, a vitamin deficiency state (lack of vitamin C or P), is one of the acquired hemorrhagic angiopathies, presenting checkerboard petechiae on nutmeg grater-like follicular hyperkeratoses, and also subperiosteal or gingival bleeding. At present this disease

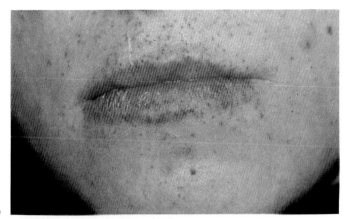

Fig. 230. Osler's disease

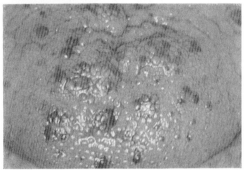

Fig. 231. Osler's disease of the
tongue

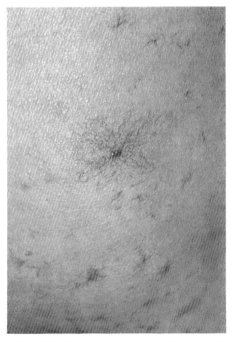

Fig. 232. Nevus araneus (spider nevus)

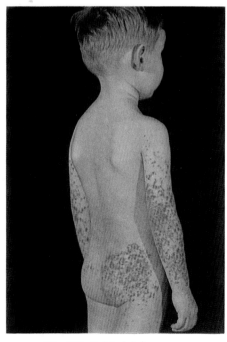

Fig. 233. Schönlein's purpura

is rarely seen in the Northern hemisphere. The most frequently acquired vascular hemorrhagic diathesis of children and adolescents is Schönlein's purpura; if complicated by additional renal and abdominal manifestations it is called Henoch's purpura. The lower parts of the body (purpura orthostatica) show transitory, slightly elevated, bright red erythemas which, under glass pressure, disclose intrafocal flea-bite-like, barely pinhead-sized spots. Pure petechial lesions occur in older exanthems (SCHÖNLEIN). Pathogenesis and pathologic anatomy are those of a leukoclastic hemorrhagic microbid, characterized by recurrences and frequently rheumatoid components (SCHÖNLEIN: Peliosis rheumatica). They are caused by allergies to infections, foods, or drugs. Later autoimmune reactions may take place in protracted cases and become manifest as Waldenström's purpura hyperglobulinemica (KORTING and ADAM). Schönlein's purpura with abdominal and renal manifestations, observed chiefly in children, may have vital consequences, because renal purpura with diapedesis of red blood cells can develop into diffuse glomerulonephritis, occasionally leading to uremic precoma. Since it is more or less refractory to steroids, the outcome may be fatal.

The most severe form of cutaneous *anaphylactoid purpura*, resembling the Sanarelli-Shwartzman phenomenon, is *purpura fulminans* (HENOCH, 1884). It acutely follows scarlet fever or varicella. The absence of factor V and a surplus of antithrombin may play a causative role. Its widespread suffusions (but not the severe vascular collapse) resemble the *Waterhouse-Friderichsen syndrome*, with hemorrhages into the adrenal glands. It occurs in Neisserian meningitis or pneumococcal sepsis.

According to present opinion, vascular *purpura in cutis laxa* (Ehlers-Danlos syndrome) is caused by too much strain on blood vessels insufficiently embedded in abnormal collagen bundles.

Progressive pigmentary purpura

LEVER, as well as KALKOFF, classified a group of skin diseases presenting rusty brown, frequently annular lesions. In this group there is an unusually large variety of entities (purpura Majocchi, purpura caused by the sedative carbromal, and others). For obvious reasons these conditions are rarely seen in children. Just as rare are secondary hemorrhagic eczemas (with the exception of the thrombocytopenic Aldrich's syndrome), previously discussed in the chapter on eczema. The same is true for the appearance of purpura in cryoglobulinemia, or in states with an increase of other thermoactive serum globulins in children.

Thrombocytic disorders

Thrombasthenia (Glanzmann-Naegeli)

A multifaceted picture of Werlhof's disease with anisothrombocytosis, disturbance of agglutination, and absence of retraction of the blood platelets is seen in early childhood.

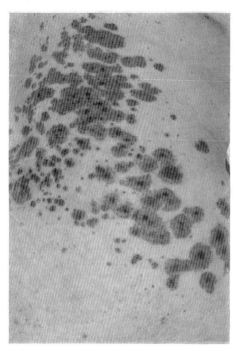

Fig. 234. Schönlein's purpura
(focal petechial hemorrhages)

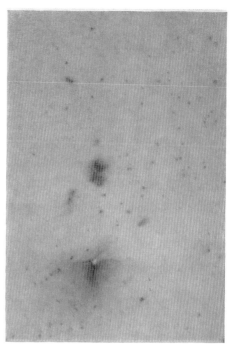

Fig. 235. Exanthem in meningococcal
infection

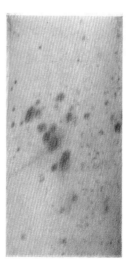

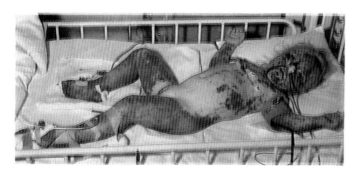

Fig. 236. Waterhouse-Friderichsen syndrome

Fig. 237. Werlhof's
purpura. Dark bluish-
red petechiae and
ecchymoses

Idiopathic thrombocytopenic purpura

In 1735, WERLHOF described the clinical manifestations of thrombocytopenia, which can occur in adolescence and, in its acute form, in childhood. Predominant is the triple syndrome of hemorrhages from all body openings (but absence of bleeding into articular spaces), petechiae, and suffusions, that is, the simultaneous presence of areas of punctate and diffuse macular bleeding. Trauma or endocrine influences (premenstruum) are additional causative factors. Laboratory tests show thrombocytopenia (without significant anemia or leukopenia), immature megakaryocytes of the bone marrow, a positive Coombs' test, as well as prolonged recalcification time, pathologic retraction of blood coagulum, and a positive Rumpel-Leede test. Splenomegaly is almost always absent. In children, acute Werlhof's disease presents as an exanthem, usually following by a few days an infection (grippe, varicella, measles, or infectious mononucleosis). In the adult, thrombocytopenia, chiefly the result of drug allergy (quinine), frequently becomes manifest within hours. The chronic type of Werlhof's disease showing a predilection for the female sex, occurs primarily between the ages of 15 and 25.

Thrombocytopenic purpura of the newborn is due to the presence of diaplacental autoaggressins of the mother suffering from essential thrombocytopenia (even without manifest cutaneous bleeding), or of other autoaggressins resulting from drug allergy, in the fetus.

The syndrome of *thrombotic-thrombocytopenic purpura*, prominent signs of which are hemolytic anemia and transitory nervous disorders, has rarely been observed in children.

Characteristics of the *Kasabach-Merritt syndrome* are giant hemangiomas with transitory thrombocytopenic purpura analogous to the purpura seen in splenic anemia. When these hemangiomas regress, either spontaneously or under treatment, thrombocytopenic purpura may become manifest (see chapter on angiomas).

Hemophilia

The hereditary coagulopathic hemorrhagic diatheses are caused by dysproteinemia or enzymatic disorders.

Their main representative is the recessively inherited sex-linked (X-chromosomal) disease called *hemophilia* by SCHÖNLEIN (1828). In hemophilia A the disturbance of coagulation is due to the deficiency of factor VIII. The smallest trauma may cause bleeding, occasionally from the umbilical cord or other locations in the first few days of life. Later when walking is attempted there may be hemorrhages into skin, muscles, and joints (hemarthrosis) with varying degrees of severity.

Hemophilia B (Christmas disease, PTC deficiency) is clinically identical, but here the deficiency of factor IX is responsible.

Parahemophilia is caused by factor V deficiency; clinically it scarcely differs from hemophilia.

Many coagulopathias are due to disturbances of the blood clotting mechanism. Textbooks on hematology should be consulted for details. From a pediatric point of view, lack of fibrinogen, or a factor I defect, should be mentioned, since it causes such a severe hemorrhagic diathesis (bleeding from the umbilical cord and into the brain) that the patient usually dies from this dominantly inherited disease at an early age.

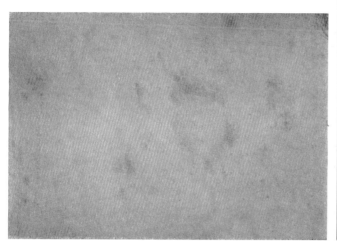

Fig. 238. Progressive pigmentary purpura (appearing here as purpura annularis Majocchi)

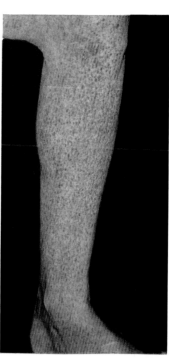

Fig. 239. Werlhof's purpura

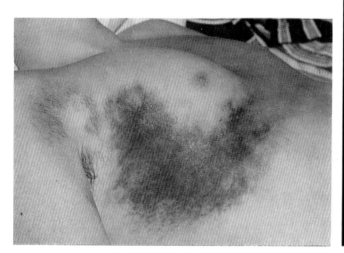

Fig. 240. Hemophilia

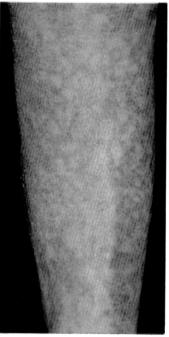

Fig. 241. Progressive pigmentary purpura (in a boy after prolonged use of sleeping pills)

Coagulopathias with prolonged clotting and normal bleeding time manifest, upon minor provocation, large areas of bleeding that is difficult to stop. The skin shows flat or hematoma-like elevated suffusions. Punctate bleeding, on the other hand, points to thrombopathic or vascular hemorrhagic diatheses. The coagulopathias become manifest at an early age or at puberty. In later life the hemorrhagic tendency frequently becomes less pronounced.

19. Metabolic and Storage Diseases

Porphyrias

Porphyrins (HOPPE-SEYLER) are quantitatively changed in cases of increased excretion of normal porphyrins, that is, in *porphyrinurias* (resulting from lead intoxication, sleeping pills, or secondary to liver disease); they are qualitatively altered in the genetically determined inborn errors of metabolism of red blood cell formation, with the excretion of porphyrins that are normally not present, as seen in the *porphyrias*. Porphyria presents gastrointestinal, neuropsychiatric, and, most important, cutaneous symptoms in various degrees of severity, according to the underlying porphyrin disorder.

Hydroa aestivale, or *"summer prurigo"* (HUTCHINSON), is a mild, hydroa vacciniforme (BAZIN, 1861), which occurs in the first years of life or sometimes around puberty. In this serious dermatosis, light-exposed areas of the skin present first clear but later cloudy vesiculo-bullous lesions, which become crusted and (especially in hydroa vacciniforme) heal with scar formation. Porphyrinuria may be present or absent. The majority of these somewhat dissimilar entities, which were formerly grouped together as hydroas, belong to the chronic polymorphous light eruptions; others belong to the porphyrias.

The porphyrias are divided into two main groups, the hepatic and the erythropoietic types.

Hepatic porphyrias

Important in this group is *porphyria hepatica acuta intermittens*, which is either a dominantly inherited enzymatic defect of the liver cells or an entity caused by toxic factors and showing precursors of porphyrin in the urine (porphobilinogen and delta-amino levulinic acid). With the exception of melanodermas, there are no cutaneous manifestations. The "acute abdomen," polyneuritic or cerebral symptoms, and also Korsakoff-like symptoms are predominant. For quick orientation, Ehrlich's aldehyde reaction in reverse is used (red discoloration results when a few drops of urine are added to several cc. of reagent). The Watson-Schwartz modification of the Ehrlich reaction may also be used. It gives the following immediate result: When chloroform is added to a positive Ehrlich test it will turn red owing to the presence of urobilinogen; porphyrin, however, will not.

Porphyria cutanea tarda (WALDENSTRÖM) or *hepatica* (WATSON). This dermatosis with actinic traumatic bullous lesions begins rather late, rarely before the age of 50 or 60. There is a tendency to diabetes and hypersideremia with lack of transferrin, formation of bullae with subsequent development of milia, hypertrichosis, melanodermas, and occasionally sclerovitiligenous areas and partial red-green color blindness. Men having outdoor occupations and alcoholics are primarily affected.

South African porphyria (porphyria variegata). In porphyria variegata we observe the same cutaneous changes seen in porphyria cutanea tarda, with marked susceptibility of the skin to mechanical insults on light-exposed areas. At the same time there are symptoms of acute intermittent porphyria. The disease appears around puberty.

Erythropoietic porphyrias

To this group belongs "*porphyria congenita*," which, according to WALDENSTRÖM, is an "avis rarissima," because only a hundred cases at the most have been observed. The tendency to this disease is recessively inherited with the presence of Type 1 porphyrins, and the disease begins in early childhood (rarely after the sixth year); there is burgundy red urine (diapers are stained red) and extreme sensitivity to light with formation of bullae (hydroa aestivale, or others), followed by ulceration and shrinking scars, especially of the nose, ears, and fingers (sclerodactylia). Additional findings are alopecia, dirty gray skin, atrophy, and loss of nails. An important sign is erythrodontia. The deciduous teeth show reddish-brown to yellow staining of the enamel with fluorescence under Wood's light; the permanent teeth show deposits of porphyrin in the dentin only. In differential diagnosis, absorption of tetracycline has to be considered. Frequently red fluorescence of some of the red blood cells (porphyrocytes) can be observed. Sometimes hemolytic anemia occurs.

Familial protoporphyrinemic photodermatosis (urticaria due to light). This comparatively rare photodermatosis was first described by KOSENOW and TREIBS (1953) and later more extensively by LANGHOF (1960). Early in childhood exposure to the sun causes reddish-brown wheals or bullae on an early erythema; later colloid milia develop. A second type of this milder variety of erythropoietic protoporphyria is light urticaria of cholinergic origin. In contradistinction to "porphyria congenita" (GÜNTHER), excretion of uroporphyrin of isomer Type 1 and mutilations are absent. A short lasting fluorescence of erythrocytes and tissue sections due to increased production of protoporphyrin is, however, characteristic. In addition, there probably are deviations from the normal patterns of amino acid secretion in the urine.

Congenital erythropoietic coproporphyria. HEILMEYER and CLOTTON first observed this photodermatosis, which starts in childhood with pruritus and cutaneous swelling upon exposure to light. There are no permanent cutaneous changes, no erythrodontia, and no red discoloration of the urine. The chief sign is an extreme increase of coproporphyrin III in the erythrocytes but not in the urine or feces.

The so-called Hartnup syndrome (DENT, 1956) is caused by an enzymatic defect of tryptophane metabolism. It is inherited in a recessive manner, and presents a pellagroid photodermatosis. mental retardation, intermittent cerebellar ataxia with increased excretion of certain amino acids, indol compounds, but not porphyrins.

Lipoidoses

Lipoid storage diseases result from genetically determined enzymatic defects which cause the accumulation and storage of starter or intermediate products, which are present before the enzymatic block is operating. In the plasma, lipids in the form of lipoproteins are linked to certain protein particles belonging to the globulins. One distinguishes beta-lipoproteins containing triglycerides and a group of beta-proteins containing cholesterol-phospholipids.

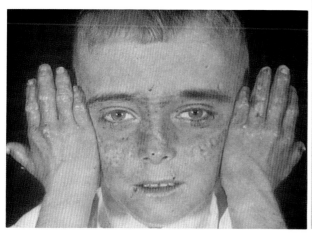

Fig. 242. Congenital porphyria

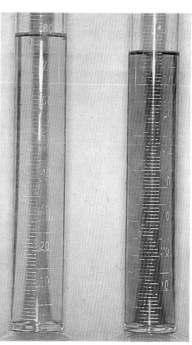

Fig. 244. Urine containing
porphyrin (right)

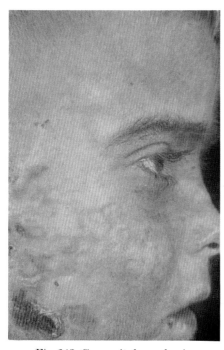

Fig. 243. Congenital porphyria

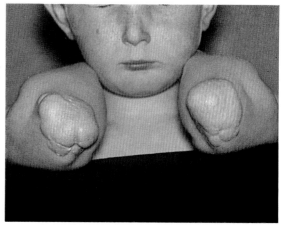

Fig. 245. Xanthomatosis

143

THANNHAUSER established the following clinical entities. *Hypercholesterolemic xanthomatosis:* The most prominent cutaneous lesions here are plane, papular, or tuberous xanthomas of characteristic yellow to reddish color, found chiefly on the eyelids. Formation of xanthomas takes place principally in mesenchymal tissue rich in mucopolysaccharides. Therefore xanthomas of tendons (Achilles, patellar, or extensor tendons of the hands) are not rare. The accompanying neutral fats in the serum are only slightly increased. One frequently observes a lipoid arcus senilis or gerontoxon, which by itself, similar to xanthoma of the eyelid, is no proof for the presence of hypercholesterolemia. Hypercholesterolemic xanthomatosis, which in most cases is transmitted in a dominant-autosomal fashion, can become vitally important because of cardiovascular involvement (of the coronary arteries and the aortic arch). Children and adolescents may die suddenly from cardiac failure when there is an abrupt heavy stress on the circulation.

Again, chiefly children and adolescents present the slowly developing lipoid gout with deposits of cholesterol symmetrically located in synovial bursae and muscles. These deposits become calcified, which leads in turn to a granulomatous lipophagia resulting in scar formation. *Xanthomatous biliary cirrhosis of the liver* (THANNHAUSER and MEGENDANTZ, 1937) is seen chiefly in older women with icteric cirrhosis, pruritus, and hypercholesterolemia.

Hyperlipemic xanthomatoses present, almost exclusively, papular and tuberous xanthomas. The serum has a creamy milky consistency. The papular lesions may erupt suddenly and often regress temporarily. BÜRGER and GRÜTZ (1932) described the main type of xanthomatosis associated with hepatosplenomegaly in children. Symptomatic hyperlipemias appear following glycogen storage disease, diabetes mellitus, pancreatitis, and nephrosis.

Normocholesterolemic xanthomatoses belong to the group of histiocytoses; these will be discussed in connection with the reticuloses.

Xanthelasma palpebrarum is a purely *cutaneous lipoidosis* which may show normal serolipid values. Rarely seen before the age of 20, it occurs chiefly after the fourth decade. At a more advanced age such xanthelasmas may show comedones or cysts (xanthelasma sebaceum, HUTCHINSON).

Necrobiosis lipoidica (OPPENHEIM, 1929; URBACH, 1932) presents almost exclusively on both legs, more often with single than multiple scleroderma-like infiltrates with telangiectases on the surface and later a mildly depressed ivory-yellow center. We have seen this condition repeatedly in adolescents; it is seldom observed in children, and occurs chiefly in diabetic or latent diabetic women between the ages of 20 and 40.

Nevoxanthoendothelioma is considered by some to be another cutaneous lipoidosis. It is the type of xanthoma most frequently seen in children. Occasionally inner organs (liver, lungs, and testes) are affected. This condition is therefore close to Hand-Schüller-Christian disease.

144

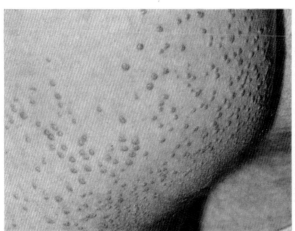

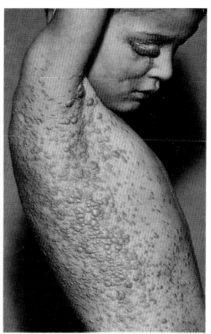

Fig. 246. Papular eruptive xanthomas of buttocks   Fig. 247. Xanthomatosis

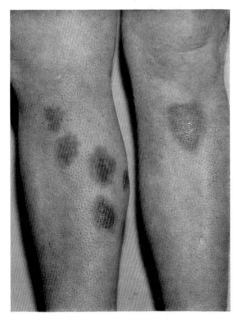

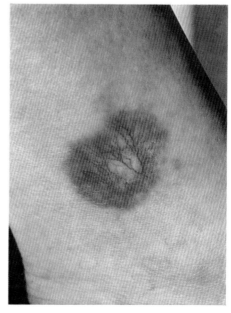

Fig. 248. Necrobiosis lipoidica

Fig. 249. Necrobiosis lipoidica
(solitary lesion)

The histology represents a type of histiocytoma; however, in the strict sense, histiocytomas will hardly regress spontaneously, in contrast to the nevoxanthoendothelioma. Nevoxantho-endothelioma appears mainly on the face, especially toward the hairline, in children up to the second year of life. The lesions are up to 1.0 cm. in size, are single or multiple, semispherical, yellowish, comparatively soft, and nonulcerated.

Amyloidosis

The fibril-forming cell product *amyloid* (VIRCHOW) may be deposited between cells, on circumscribed areas, and perireticularly or around connective tissue. It may occur as a generalized amyloidosis, as well. Such deposits, which are more frequently observed in older people, can be acquired (as in secondary amyloidosis), can be inherited, or may occur as an idiopathic primary amyloidosis. The presence of amyloid is proved by microscopic examination under polarized light (congo red) or fluorescence (thioflavine). Acquired pericollagenous amyloidoses are found chiefly in plasmocytoma or macroglobulinemia. The main signs of familial amyloidosis are renal disease, neuropathy, and myocardial involvement. Twenty-five per cent of patients suffering from generalized amyloidosis present cutaneous changes with petechiae, suffusions, papulo-lichenoid lesions, subcutaneous infiltrations, scleroderma-like manifestations, or poikiloderma-like lesions. Localized cutaneous amyloidosis may resemble neurodermatitis circumscripta or, may, on the legs, suggest prurigo (lichen amyloidosus).

Hyalinosis cutis et mucosae (lipoid proteinosis)

Clinically, this disease resembles paramyloidosis with a PAS-positive (WEYBRECHT and KORTING) substance probably derived from the blood and composed of phospholipids and glucoproteins. Deposits of this substance may cause hoarseness at birth or in the first months of life, followed by slowly progressive but still reversible cutaneous changes of the face, head, axillae, or acra. Nodular, hyperkeratotic, yellowish-white to brownish, sometimes verrucous lesions, are associated with white atrophic areas. Macroglossia with loss of papillary ridges is also seen in this storage disease. Medically important are involvement of the esophagus and stomach and the presence of intracranial areas of calcification. This disease is apparently transmitted as an autosomal recessive characteristic. Isolated cases have been seen after scarlet fever, diphtheria, or smallpox inoculation.

Mucinosis

In contrast to diffuse genuine myxedema, which is seen primarily in women between the fourth and fifth decades, but also in children (cretinism), the abortive localized lesions of mucinosis (circumscribed pretibial myxedema usually in connection with hyperthyroidism, RICHTER, KEINING), and the euthyroid myxodermias (lichen myxedematosus, NEUMANN, 1935, or scleromyxedema complicated by paraproteinemia, ARNDT-GOTTRON), are found only in older age groups.

146

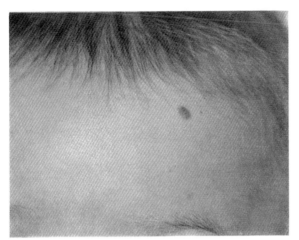

Fig. 250. Nevoxanthoendothelioma

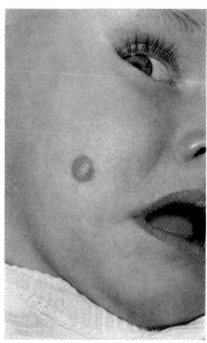

Fig. 251. Nevoxanthoendothelioma

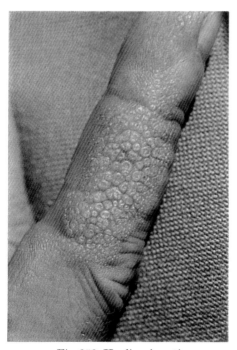

Fig. 252. Hyalinosis cutis

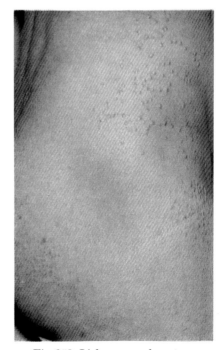

Fig. 253. Lichen myxedematosus

147

Sphingolipidoses (Niemann-Pick disease, Gaucher's disease)

While cutaneous lesions are absent in Tay-Sachs disease, Niemann-Pick disease presents melanin pigmentations, occasionally resembling mongolian spots, and less frequently xanthomas or erysipelas-like or granulomatous infiltrates. The skin manifestations of Gaucher's disease consist chiefly of melanin pigmentations, purpuric exanthems, or uncharacteristic ecthymas.

Cutaneous gout

Primary chronic cutaneous gout (usually in the form of butter-cream colored tophi on the rims of the ears or the tips of the fingers) usually affects males after the age of 40; however, GOTTRON and KORTING once observed multiple small tophi which had been present on the fingers since the twentieth year of life.

Calcinosis cutis

Deposition of calcium salts in the skin or subcutaneous tissue may appear in metastatic form (VIRCHOW), that is, in systemic disturbances of calcium and phosphorus metabolism (vitamin D intoxication, the milk and alkali syndrome) or in metabolic form (with normal blood calcium and phosphorus values) in scleroderma (THIBIÈRGE and WEISSENBACH, 1911) or dermatomyositis (RUDOLPH, 1934). Localized disturbances of circulation also seem to be of occasional importance for the calcium deposits. The term *dystrophic calcinosis* is used to describe calcification of previously damaged tissue (for example, in pseudoxanthoma elasticum, in Malherbe's calcifying epithelioma, or in the Ehlers-Danlos syndrome). In the absence of an underlying systemic disease, such as juvenile dermatomyositis, children with metastatic calcinosis may present general lymphadenopathy, anemia, increase in gamma globulin, and also hepatosplenomegaly.

Ochronosis

Alkaptonuria, described in a 44 year old diabetic in 1859 by BÖDIKER, was the first known example of recessive inheritance in man. In 1891 WOLKOW and BAUMANN found homogentisic acid to be its chemical substrate. Before this, however, VIRCHOW spoke in 1866 of the "ochronosis of the cartilage and bony-like structures."

In early infancy the darkening of diapers indicates the presence of homogentisic acid in the urine. The conspicuous brownish or bluish deposition of pigment (on the sclerae or the ears) or the ochronosis of the cartilage may begin as late as around the thirtieth or fortieth years. At this time homogentisic acid is no longer fully excreted in the urine. The patient suffering from ochronosis may present a cicatrizing alopecia and diminished intelligence.

Pseudoalkaptonuria has been observed after external application of phenol, pyrogallol (pyrogallic acid), or beechwood tar.

Alkaptonuria is caused by the absence of an enzyme in the metabolism of phenylalanine and tyrosine, and can be recognized by examining the urine with TROMMER's or FEHLING's tests, paper chromatography, or by the addition of ferric chloride, which produces an evanescent blue or green discoloration.

148

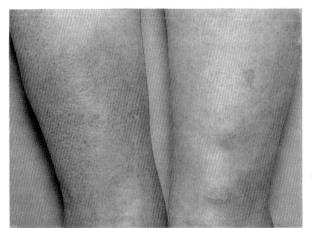

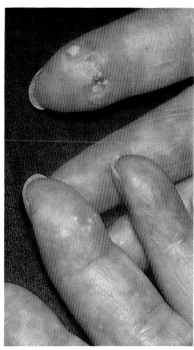

Fig. 254. Circumscribed pretibial myxedema (in a young woman)

Fig. 255. Cutaneous gout (in a young woman)

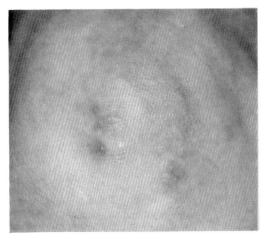

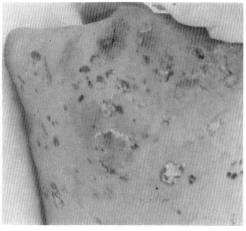

Fig. 256. Calcinosis cutis

Fig. 257. Calcinosis cutis (with discharging concrements)

Phenylketonuria

In 1934 Fölling first described phenylpyruvic oligophrenia, a disease which becomes manifest shortly after birth. The cutaneous changes are not characteristic: delicate skin, tendency to diminished pigmentation, eczematous changes, follicular keratoses, hyperhidrosis, photosensitivity, and others. The disease is transmitted by an autosomal recessive gene. The diagnosis is made by the dark blue-green color that develops when 10 per cent ferric chloride solution is added to acidified urine, or by the "phenistix-test."

Recently, the Guthrie test has been used, because the urine of older children frequently does not react to the ferric chloride test. (This happens when the blood level of phenylalanine is below 20 mg. per 100 ml.)

Carotinosis

The young child with carotinosis presents a distinctive yellow discoloration of the palms and soles, and occasionally a systemic involvement (sparing the conjunctiva) as well. It is caused by eating foods containing carotene or lycopene (an isomer of beta-carotene). In the adult carotinosis is also determined by the level of the serum lipids. Even without an excessive intake of carotene it may develop in diabetes, hyperthyroidism, or nephrosis. Yellow discoloration of the palms and soles is also seen in typhoid and pellagra.

Angiokeratoma corporis diffusum

Since Fabry's description of cutaneous lesions which appear as widespread dark blue to blackish, barely keratotic papules (in contrast to the name "angiokeratoma") measuring a few millimeters in diameter (Steiner and Voerner, angiomatosis miliaris), the present concept of angiokeratoma has evolved to embrace a cardiovasorenal syndrome (Ruiter-Pompen). It is considered to be a sphingosintrihexosid or ceramidetrihexosid thesaurismosis (or a ceramidetrihexosidase deficiency). The cutaneous lesions favor the central portions of the trunk, especially the umbilical region, but spare the palms, the soles, and the face. The lips may also be involved. Some of the patients present disturbances of sweat secretion, fever, cardiomegaly, cerebrovascular signs, lipoidosis of the cornea, microhematuria, and proteinuria with excretion of double refractive substances ("Maltese crosses"). As a rule, this storage disease favors the male sex; it becomes manifest around the seventh to eighth years of life, or later.

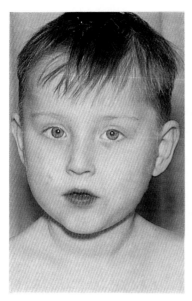

Fig. 258. Light complexion in
phenylketonuria

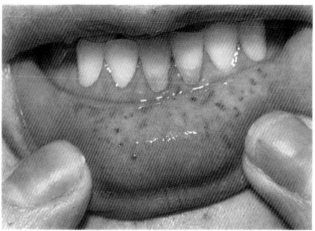

Fig. 259. Angiokeratoma corporis diffusum (Fabry's disease)

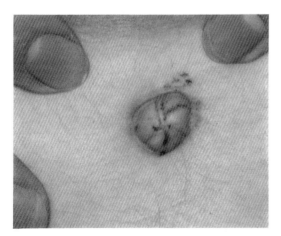

Fig. 260. Angiokeratoma corporis diffusum
(Typical localization on umbilicus)

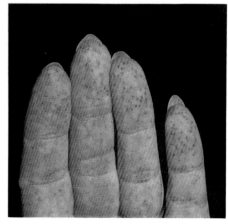

Fig. 261. Angiokeratoma corporis
diffusum

20. Collagenosis Group (Generalized Connective Tissue Diseases)

The following disease entities, which will – not without opposition – be discussed together, differ in site, age, sex, course, and also the nature of cutaneous lesions. Important in acute *lupus erythematosus* are autoimmune processes. Circumscribed and especially progressive *scleroderma* may constitute a neurovascularly induced disease process with decisive pathogenic effects on the different collagen fractions. *Dermatomyositis* is based on a disturbed enzyme mechanism, probably due to a change of the permeability of the vascular endothelium. Of these three systemic diseases, dermatomyositis occurs most frequently in childhood (about 20 per cent of all cases are observed in patients below the age of 15). The association of the dermatoses with internal malignancies, so important in later life, is uncommon at an early age. Therefore the prognosis of dermatomyositis in childhood is much more favorable. Nevertheless, there is a tendency to contractures and metabolic calcium deposits in the soft parts of the extremities.

Dermatomyositis

The diagnosis of dermatomyositis is currently based upon skin and muscle biopsies, the determination of urinary creatine and creatinine (in childhood they may be present physiologically), an electromyogram, and chiefly the determination of the enzymes SGOT, SGPT, aldolase, creatinephosphokinase (CPK) and myokinase. As mentioned before, it is important to consider a possible underlying disease (malignant tumor, rheumatic disease, tuberculosis), the significance of light sensitivity, temperature changes (especially exposure to severe cold), and different external injurious agents. This disease was already known in the last century. In 1930 GOTTRON studied it extensively. The acute case shows peculiar heliotrope, wine-red to reddish-violet (rarely whitish), later telangiectatic or speckled, lesions which, on the back of the neck, may be interspersed with lichenoid papules.

152

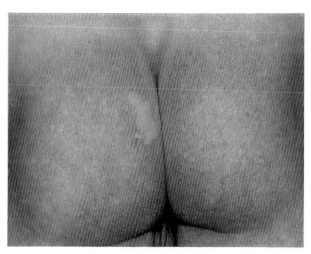

Fig. 264. Dermatomyositis

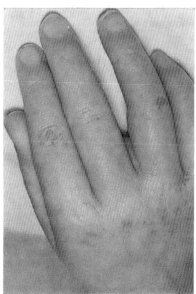

Fig. 263. Dermatomyositis

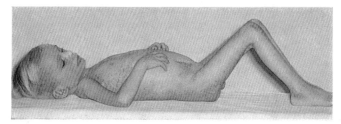

Fig. 262. Dermatomyositis

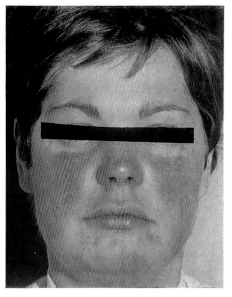

Fig. 265. Subacute lupus erythematosus

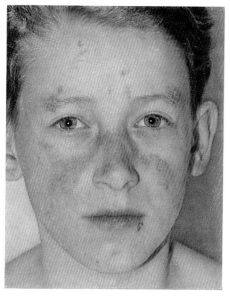

Fig. 266. Subacute lupus erythematosus

Poikiloderma may represent the final stage of dermatomyositis, presenting a triad of atrophy, pigmentation, and telangiectases. JACOBI (1906) called attention to this dermatosis, naming it *poikiloderma atrophicans vasculare*. In rare cases it may be congenital or occur in early childhood, and may be associated with a variety of congenital defects. In ROTHMUND's and THOMSON's syndromes of congenital dystrophy, poikiloderma is associated with the formation of cataracts, dystrophy of the nails, hypogonadism, and premature arteriosclerosis. Poikiloderma of the type Zinsser (1906) or Cole, Rauschkolb, and Toomey (1930) presents reticulated or neviform pigmentations, atrophy, dystrophic fingernails and toenails, marked leukokeratoses, and hyperhidrosis. Also to be mentioned are the dwarfs described first by BLOOM and later by KORTING, ADAM, and others with congenital telangiectatic lupus erythematosus-like cutaneous changes.

Lupus erythematosus

According to today's knowledge lupus erythematosus is based on widespread changes of the connective tissue of the blood vessels, with excessive reactivity (hyperergy) to streptococcal infections (pharyngitis, antistreptolysin titer above 600 units). There is a genetic disposition to formation of unusual pathologic immune bodies (lupus erythematosus cells, hematoxylin bodies). There also exist lupus erythematosus-like conditions caused by hydralazine (Apresoline), griseofulvin, tetracycline, hydantoin, and chlorpromazine (Aphenothiazine). Splenectomy may also contribute to such conditions.

Chronic discoid or cutaneous lupus erythematosus of the face presents follicular erythema, follicular hyperkeratosis (carpet-tack phenomenon), follicular and finally macular atrophies, primarily in butterfly distribution. Sometimes the pinna of the ears and the terminal parts of the extremities are affected, as in the so-called "Chilblain-lupus" (HUTCHINSON). In multisystemic visceral acute lupus erythematosus we find discrete cutaneous changes with petechial bleeding intrafocally and also on mucous membranes, with simultaneous marked constitutional signs. There is involvement of the lymph nodes, joints, serous membranes (polyserositis), and nonbacterial verrucous inflammation of the valves, the endocardium (KAPOSI, 1872; LIBMAN and SACHS, 1924), and the kidneys, with histologically characteristic wire-loop lesions. The lesions are formed by deposits of a homogenous, eosinophilic substance in the thickened basal membranes of the glomeruli, the eyegrounds, and the nervous system.

Scleroderma

Localized and progressive scleroderma

"Real" progressive scleroderma is extremely rare in childhood. Our own observations are lacking. Systemic involvement, with progressive scleroderma, has been seen in children. This systemic disease of the blood vessels and connective tissue has the attributes of a fatal disorder (fibrosis of the myocardium, pulmonary sclerosis, gastrointestinal slowing of passage with constipation, eventually ending in fatal paralytic ileus). The disease starts characteristically as a vasomotoric acrodermatosis (acrosclerosis, later also sclerodactylia), with Ray-

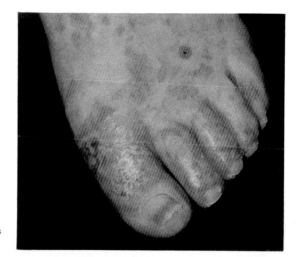

Fig. 267. Subacute lupus erythematosus
("chilblain" lupus)

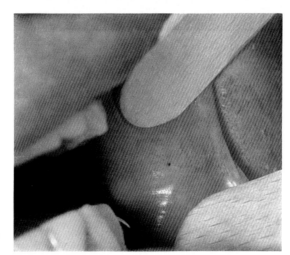

Fig. 268. Subacute lupus erythematosus.
Petechiae of oral mucosa

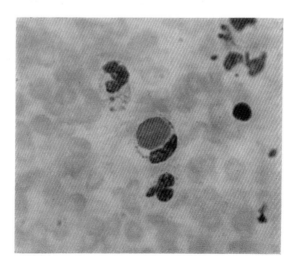

Fig. 269. Lupus erythematosus cell

naud-like changes. *Localized scleroderma* is, without question, more frequent in young children, representing a transitory disease with spontaneous involution. Three main types may be seen: linear morphea ("en bandes," "en coup de sabre"), scleroderma in plaques, and small subacute erythematous macules of a rose to faded yellow-red color, surrounded in characteristic fashion by the so-called lilac ring. Such areas of morphea may persist for years before their final involution sets in. Bandlike scleroderma of the extremities, occurring in childhood and chiefly in girls, develops more slowly and involutes to a lesser degree than the other two types. It may interfere with the growth of the affected extremity.

Lichen sclerosus and atrophicus

This disease differs from the small macular type of localized scleroderma (both may occur in grouped single lesions) by its more grayish-white color, in comparison with the milky-butter shade of small macular morphea, and also by the infrequent presence of follicular hyperkeratoses within the lesions. In addition, the single lesions are less indurated, and according to their atrophic character they present delicate atrophic folds with a suggestion of a dirty-brown hyperpigmented margin. Sites of predilection, sometimes even in young children, are the vulva and the perianal region.

Scleredema adultorum (Buschke, 1900)

In many respects this disease closely resembles HARDY'S (1877) "edematous scleroderma." It is essentially a mucopolysaccharide thesaurismosis, that is, a kind of systemic storage disease. Observations of patients so far reveal that the disorder tends to occur slightly more frequently in females. Patients tend to be under the age of 20. Characteristic is the onset of the disorder after an infectious disease, the absence of manifestations on the distal parts of the extremities, especially the hands, and the definite tendency to spontaneous involution, chiefly in children. The skin has a waxy or paraffin-like consistency. These changes are more palpable than visible. The cutaneous surface may be nodular, wavily trabecular, or furrowed.

Scleroderma-like diseases of childhood

Sclerema neonatorum. Formerly, this peculiar diffuse induration of the skin and subcutaneous tissue was often called "scleroderma of infants." One has always distinguished between *sclerema edematosum* and *sclerema adiposum*, the fat sclerema, in which finger pressure will not result in pitting of the skin, as it will in scleredema edematosum. In spite of this supposed difference in the character of the edema, both pathologic conditions show the same alabaster to yellowish-white or marble-like hue. At the periphery the color tends to be cyanotic. Although the surface of the diseased area is smooth, it is sometimes uneven or interspersed with palpable nodules or cystic formations in the deeper portions. It is important to differentiate other forms of edema occurring in the newborn (Rh incompatibility, hypoproteinemia due to pancreatic fibrosis, and similar conditions).

156

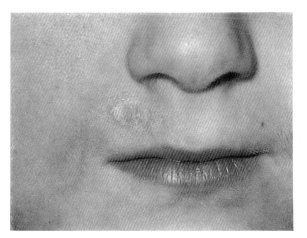

Fig. 270. Circumscribed scleroderma (Morphea)

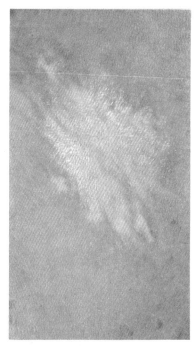

Fig. 271. Circumscribed
scleroderma en plaques

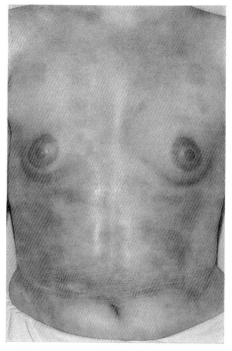

Fig. 273. Circumscribed scleroderma
(widespread)

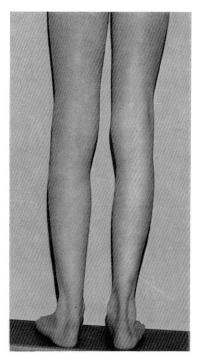

Fig. 272. Circumscribed
scleroderma en bandes
(smallness of the right leg)

Subcutaneous fat necrosis of the newborn or adiponecrosis subcutanea neonatorum. This frequently symmetric fat sclerosis in newborn babies was formerly misdiagnosed as "infantile scleroderma." Its plaque-like subcutaneous indurations are located mainly on the back, buttocks, cheeks, or extremities. The disease chiefly affects overweight babies who were born after difficult labor and are apparently in excellent general health. The induration can be moved very little from its base. The sharply circumscribed deep-seated plaques are demarcated like epaulets. The overlying skin is frequently brownish or bluish-red in color. Sometimes septic softening intervenes; otherwise involution ensues after months, with insignificant residual lipoatrophy. This idiopathic disease of the subcutaneous fat of the infant represents decomposition of the fat into anisotropic fats, causing granulomatous proliferations.

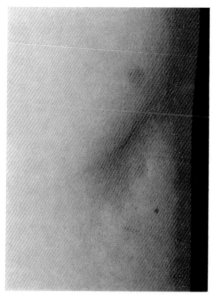

Fig. 274. Healed localized
scleroderma with trough-like
depression ("localized panatrophy")

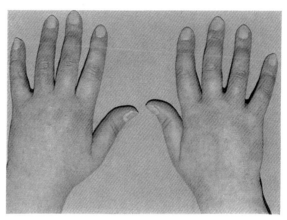

Fig. 275. Raynaud's syndrome (beginning progressive
scleroderma)

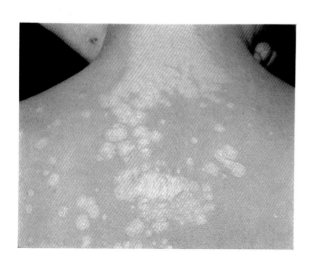

Fig. 276. Lichen sclerosus et atrophicus

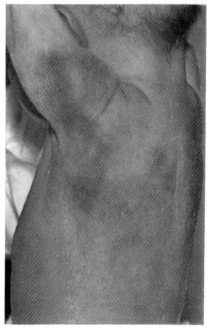

Fig. 277. Subcutaneous fat necrosis

21. Atrophies of the Skin

Cutaneous atrophy is a regression which fundamentally represents aging of the tissue and is therefore observed in later stages of life. *Atrophic striae distensae* of the skin, however, occur exclusively in young people. They present as occasionally depressed and later ruffled distended streaks which are first reddish-blue, later more bluish-gray, and finally mother-of-pearl colored. The *striae of puberty* occur predominantly on the buttocks and thighs. Systemic cortisone therapy results as frequently in striae as local cortisone injections result in atrophy.

Atrophodermia vermiculata (DARIER), which is a cutaneous atrophy of neviform character, commonly starts in prepuberty but may appear in infancy. Peculiar netlike lesions with dilated follicles and the formation of pseudocomedones give the skin a worm-eaten appearance. It is limited almost exclusively to the zygomatic region.

Macular atrophy, or dermatitis maculosa atrophicans, is primarily a disease of the young. It occurs primarily in females. *Anetoderma erythematosa* (THIBIÈRGE, JADASSOHN) begins with inflammatory macules. Anetoderma of the Pellizzari type is diagnosed when macular atrophy develops at the site of a preceding urticarial lesion. The Schweninger-Buzzi type presents saccular or hernia-like protrusions with increased volume above the level of the skin.

160

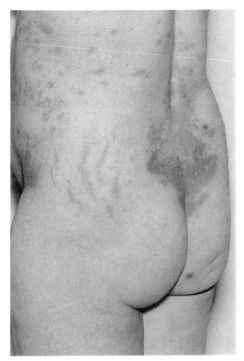

Fig. 278. Striae after systemic cortisone therapy

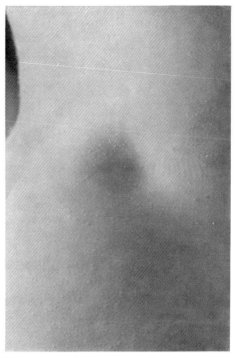

Fig. 279. Localized panatrophy at the site of repository cortisone injection

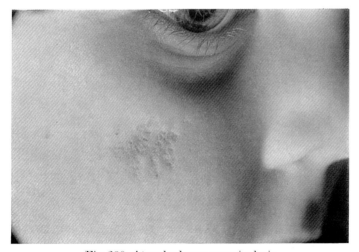

Fig. 280. Atrophoderma vermicularis

Although *acrodermatitis chronica atrophicans* (BUCHWALD, HERXHEIMER and HARTMANN) is quite frequently observed in younger people, it unquestionably favors women in the fifth or sixth decade of life. This slowly developing atrophy of one or several extremities starts with lymphohistiocytic or edematous-infiltrative (PICK: erythromelia) changes, which later develop into flaccid-atrophic, and more rarely into scleroderma-like, hard, atrophic changes, with transparency of the larger deeper veins. Occasionally, fibroid juxta-articular nodules, similar to those observed in proven treponematoses, are seen. In spite of this, acrodermatitis atrophicans apparently is not a treponematosis, although there have been isolated observations of spirochetes in the tissue, isolated positive results of the pallida serum reaction, and an unequivocal response of the disease to penicillin in the preatrophic stage. Changes in regional lymph nodes and bone marrow, an increased sedimentation rate, and also the frequently associated macrocryoglobulinemia speak in favor of a systemic disease, originally caused by an infectious agent (transmitted by ticks ?). Newer transplantation experiments may support this view.

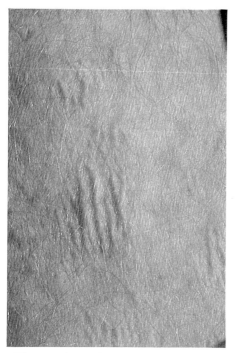

Fig. 281. Anetoderma (Jadassohn type)

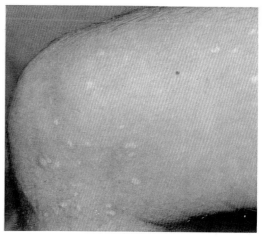

Fig. 282. Anetoderma (Schweninger-Buzzi type)

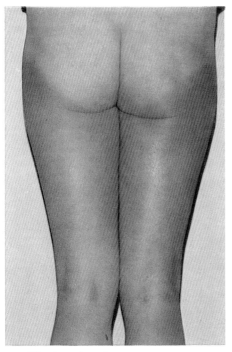

Fig. 283. Acrodermatitis chronica
atrophicans (early, edematous,
infiltrative stage)

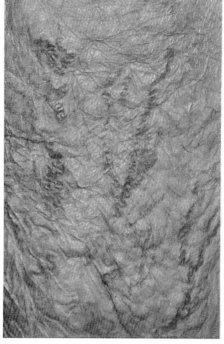

Fig. 284. Acrodermatitis chronica
atrophicans (flaccid atrophic end stage in
an adult woman)

22. Avitaminosis

At the present time diseases caused by a relative lack of one or several vitamins (poly-hypovitaminoses) are rarely seen. Even complex avitaminoses are rarely the result of a nutritional deficiency but more likely the result of a metabolic defect. The most prominent sign of *vitamin A avitaminosis* is phrynoderma (NICHOLLS), or toadskin. In addition, night blindness and xerosis (BITOT, 1832) may be seen. These two conditions cannot always be strictly differentiated from vitamin C deficiency. Toadskin is composed of sometimes localized, follicular keratotic papules, which are more prevalent at sites of pressure. Together with dryness (xerosis) of the integument, a peculiar ashy gray or brownish-gray discoloration should lead one to suspect the etiologic possibility of the lack of vitamin A. A similar cutaneous aspect of folliculo-keratotic and ichthyosiform lesions is found in *vitamin C deficiency;* such a "lichen scorbuticus" prepares the groundwork for follicular scorbutic bleeding arranged in a chessboard pattern. With further exacerbation there follow cutaneous petechiae, hemorrhages, or internal bleeding into body cavities. The suffusions of scurvy prefer areas of special muscular stress, such as the popliteal spaces and the subcutis of the tibiae. Palpation of such hematomas results in reflex-like contractions of the involved muscular areas. HEUBNER called this "the puppet string phenomenon." Patients in possession of their teeth will develop redness and spongy, dusky red swelling of the interdental papillae, especially of the incisors. In infants, in addition to pseudoparalysis and painful swellings of the limbs, subperiosteal hematomas (cephal hematomas), hematurias (reddish discoloration of diapers soaked with urine), or melena is observed. This infantile scurvy of the type of Möller-Barlow disease is seen chiefly during the second half of the first year of life, particularly during the winter months.

In our latitudes, vitamin B_1 deficiencies (beri-beri) are rarely observed, with the exception of ariboflavinoses of the adult (especially the diabetic). Pellagra is characterized by the four d's (diarrhea, dermatitis, dementia, death). Cutaneous changes of pellagra, so-called pellagrosis, consist of occasionally edematous but only rarely exudative, symmetric, sharply outlined erythematous areas, which after some time assume a mahogany brown color. This is followed by thin and lamellar or flour-like desquamation, which occurs chiefly in the middle region of erythematous areas, with the result that later the originally peripheral parts present hyperkeratotic, dirty borders, especially on the medial aspects of the arms. Sites of predilection of this pellagrosis are the hands, forearms, dorsa of the feet, the neck, and the sternal region (Casal's necklace). The palmar aspects of the hands present marked yellow discoloration (Flinker's sign) simultaneously with thick keratinization. The presence of filiform lesions or folliculopapular keratoses on the nasolabial folds, similar to the seborrheic-erythematous changes of the genital region, is more likely a manifestation of ariboflavinosis. The vermilion border of the lips is sore and looks as if it is covered with lacquer. The tongue has a polymorphic appearance, being highly red or bluish-purple, somewhat resembling Möller's glossitis or the so-called beefsteak tongue. Especially characteristic of patients with pellagra is profuse salivation. Sun exposure is unquestionably the most important precipitating factor for the appearance of the cutaneous manifestations of pellagra, but in contrast to scurvy, heavy bodily exercise or infections need not be contributory. Pellagra typically starts in the "stomach" (diarrhea, cystic ileitis) and occurs seasonally with some regularity, between Easter and Whitsuntide (50 days after Easter). In the past few years we have seen adults suffering from pellagra because of alcohol abuse. Juvenile pellagra, however, which usually formed the main contingent in a severe endemic, is completely absent in West Germany.

Infantile pellagra in a somewhat different form is seen on the Gold coast and in Uganda, and also in Central and South America, Costa Rica, and Brazil; it is called Kwashiorkor (Kwashi: boy; orkor: red). Similar to CZERNY's and KELLER's dystrophy, and caused by a pure carbohydrate diet consisting only of flour, the disease is characterized primarily by edema, retarded growth, low body weight, and adipose infiltration of the liver or liver cirrhosis. The Brazilian cases do not present cirrhosis, but show heavy lipoid infiltration of the liver, along with pancreatic changes. In addition to disturbed sleep, depressions, sudden pyrexia, and so forth, important dermatologic findings are hyperemia of the oral mucous membranes, a red tongue with prominent papillae, desquamating erythemas, and depigmentations.

Pantothenic acid is apparently important for melanogenesis and copper metabolism of the hair. There have been occasional observations of delayed hair growth in malnourished children. Canities, alopecia, and achromotrichia have been considered to be due to lack of pantothenic acid (apantothenosis).

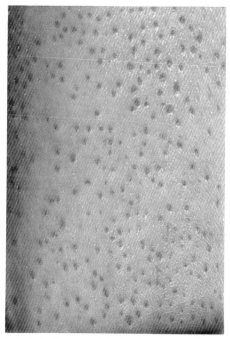

Fig. 285. Scurvy. Beginning hemorrhagic "lichen scorbuticus"

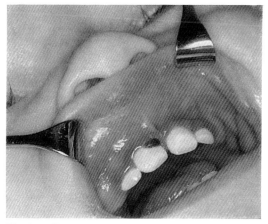

Fig. 286. Scurvy. Dusky red swelling of interdental papillae

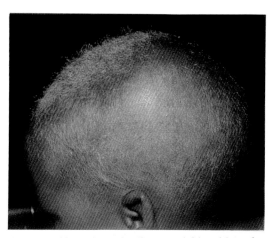

Fig. 287. Alopecia and achromotrichia of kwashiorkor

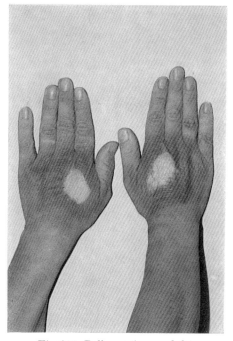

Fig. 288. Pellagra (in an adult)

167

23. Benign Tumors of the Skin

Nevi and nevoid syndromes

Nevus cell nevi, described in the chapter dealing with pigmented tumors, should not be confused with organic nevi. Nevi are cutaneous dysplasias manifest at birth or later in life. They are characterized by an excess or absence of one or more tissue components. H. PINKUS defines nevoid or organoid tumors as formations of too much immature tissue.

As examples of pigmented nevi we mention only *nevi spili* or the *flat lentigines*, which represent accumulations of pigment without nevus cells. There is a certain difference between *ephelides* (freckles) and lentigines, which show a longer or proliferating rate crest. *Syndromes with lentigines* are *Darier's lentiginosis profusa, lentiginosis centrofacialis* (TOU-RAINE), *inverse ephelides* (SIEMENS), *the association of pigmented spots and polyposis* (PEUTZ-JEGHERS, KLOSTERMANN), and the lentigo type of von Recklinghausen's disease, which belongs to the phakomatoses.

Nevus anemicus represents an irregularly outlined white spot, impressive by its negative nature and its contrast to normal or hyperpigmented skin. Its border is not hyperpigmented. After the site is rubbed the nevus becomes more conspicuous. It is not caused by lack of pigment but either by circumscribed hypoplasia of the blood vessels or their impaired faculty to dilate. Sweating and the function of the arrectores pilorum are maintained in the area of this nevus.

Phakomatoses

This concept of VAN DER HOEVE (1921) refers to a group of syndromes of anomalies which arise out of disturbances of tissue specialization in early embryonal life and continue to progress even after the embryonal period has ended. The following disorders belong to this category.

Adenoma sebaceum (Bourneville-Pringle phakomatosis; tuberous sclerosis)

In 1880 BOURNEVILLE described *tuberous sclerosis* (its main location being the area of the basal ganglia). The disorder is transmitted chiefly as a regular autosomal dominant trait. Additional hamartias are located in the eyes, kidneys, heart, and brain. The chief cutaneous change is *adenoma sebaceum* (BALZER and MENETRIER's "white variety"), or the multiple, skin-colored, symmetric, facial nevi, located chiefly in the nasolabial area. If the papules

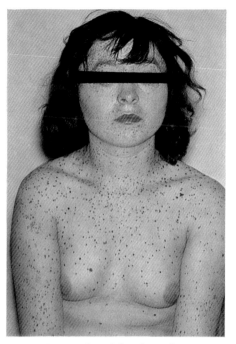

Fig. 289. Lentiginosis profusa

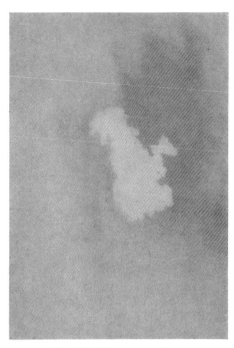

Fig. 290. Nevus anemicus

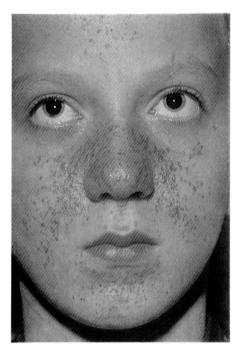

Fig. 291. Adenoma sebaceum
(Pringle's disease)

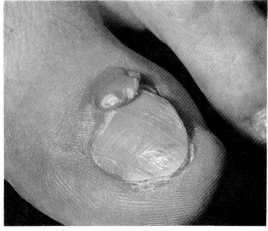

Fig. 292. Adenoma sebaceum (Koenen's periungual
tumor)

show telangiectases, the "red variety" (Pringle) is present; if extensive proliferation of the connective tissue predominates, the "hard variety" (Hallopeau and Leredde) is present. The tendency to proliferation of the connective tissue is evidenced in perigingival nodules, periungual and subungual fibromas (Koenen's tumors), and lumbosacral *shagreen patches* or *connective tissue nevi*, which usually develop as early as around the second to sixth years of life.

Von Recklinghausen's disease, neurofibromatosis

This polymorphous phakomatosis distinctly favors the male sex. Frequently present at birth, it originates in the nervous system and is caused by an autosomal dominant gene with greatly variable expressivity. Environmental factors such as pregnancies, traumas, and infectious diseases have a great influence on the course of the disorder. Manifestations such as tumors (neurinomas, neurofibromas) and macular pigmentations are found side by side. Small tumors can be pressed down but snap back in a characteristic manner. Occasionally, they are distributed along the course of a peripheral nerve. Some of the circumscribed pigmentations are large and the color of milky coffee; the small ones simulate ephelides and are of a darker tan color. If there is a group of more than six nevi spili, and especially if they happen to be located in the axillae (Crowe; axillary freckling), von Recklinghausen's disease should be suspected. Isolated manifestations of the responsible gene favor the acoustic or optic nerves, eyelids, vulva, rather frequently the gastrointestinal tract (with transitory attacks of diarrhea and abdominal pain), and the skeleton (kyphoscoliosis). Vascular neurofibromatosis is, according to Feyrter, a neurofibromatosis of the vessels, and according to Reubi, a unique vascular disease occurring in neurofibromatosis. Occasionally a neurofibroma may change into a sarcoma. Patients suffering from von Recklinghausen's disease have a dreamy, apathetic, tired, melancholic facial expression (Rille), and their physical performance is poor (they are restless and suffer from insomnia).

Pigmented spots and intestinal polyposis (Peutz-Jeghers)

This phakomatosis is most likely transmitted as an autosomal dominant. The gene shows full penetrance. Characteristically, in dark complected persons ephelis-like melanin spots are radially grouped around facial openings; there are also spots on the fingers and toes. These individuals show polyposis as well, chiefly of the small intestines (jejunum) but in rare instances also in other organs. The polyps cause intussusception, loss of blood, and secondary anemia. They become evident chiefly in the second decade, whereas the melanin spots on the oral mucosa and the lips may be present as early as at birth. The tendency of these intestinal hamartomas to become malignant is, at the present time, not considered to be high.

Melanophakomatoses

Musger considered Touraine's *melanoblastose neurocutanée*, Ota's *nevus fusco-ceruleus ophthalmo-maxillaris*, or Fitzpatrick's "oculodermal melanocytosis" to be melanophakomatoses. In the type described by Touraine, bathing suit nevi of different sizes are located

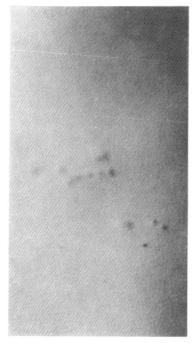

Fig. 293. Connective tissue nevi

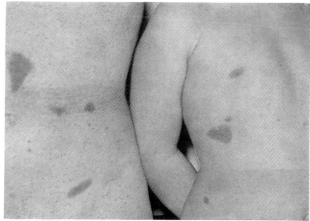

Fig. 294. Familial neurofibromatosis (von Recklinghausen's disease)

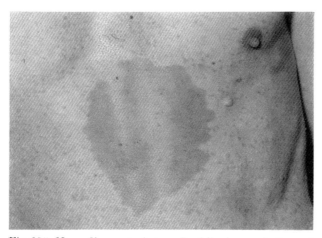

Fig. 295. Neurofibromatosis (von Recklinghausen's disease)

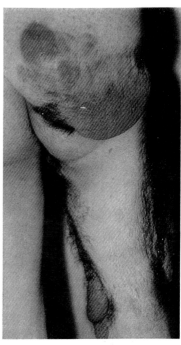

Fig. 296. von Recklinghausen's disease (paunch-like pendulous elephantiasis)

on a slightly hyperpigmented skin. They are associated with changes in the central nervous system, such as hydrocephalus, cerebral attacks, and others, but the melanin-forming tissues of the eye do not seem to take part in the process.

Epitheliomatous phakomatoses

This concept comprises early embryonal developmental disturbances such as Hermans-Herzberg's phakomatosis (MUSGER), described as nevus epitheliomatosus multiplex and also called basal cell nevus, with extremely numerous basaliomatous nodules on the skin of the trunk, face and neck, and associated with gliomas and medulloblastomas. KNOTH and EHLERS also consider Brooke's epitheliomas (pinhead- to pea-sized semiglobular, skin-colored papules on seborrheic predilection sites with onset in childhood) and the characteristic turban tumors (Spiegler's tumors with manifestations in early adulthood) to be phakomatoses.

Angiomatous phakomatoses

MUSGER considers syndromes with telangiectatic anomalies, such as the STURGE-WEBER and the KLIPPEL-TRÉNAUNAY syndromes, as belonging to the angiomatous phakomatoses. They are discussed in connection with angiomas.

Hard nevi

Solitary, hard, verrucous or hyperkeratotic nevi are rarely seen in children. Systematized nevi are observed more frequently, but these ichthyosiform, hyperkeratotic or verrucoid nevi are better termed linear dermatoses, analogously to "striated" lichen planus or lichen simplex. Such systematized nevi are symmetrically or unilaterally distributed, with unique lines and zones, but this geometric arrangement does not correspond to definite anatomic systems (nervous system, dermatomes, and so forth).

Organic nevi

The main representatives of these organic or glandular nevi, which are determined by abnormal genes, are the *nevus sebaceus* and the *sweat gland nevus*. *Nevus sebaceus* is usually present at birth and is located chiefly on the scalp, over the sutures of the skull behind the ears, or in a systematic linear arrangement. It consists of groups of about 1×3 cm. large yellow-red, closely aggregated nodules. The main representatives of the *sweat gland nevi* are the *syringomas* or *hydradenomas*, also caused by abnormal genes. These multiple hamartias affect chiefly females. They become evident late, usually after the second decade, are located on the anterior chest and eyelids, and consist of flat, pinhead to lentil-sized, moderately firm, yellow-brown, smooth nodules, most of which are present throughout life.

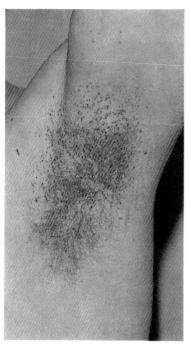

Fig. 297. Profuse axillary
lentigines (von Recklinghausen's
disease ?)

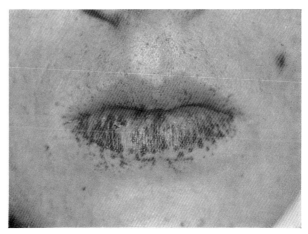

Fig. 298. Pigmented spots of the lips in Peutz-Jeghers
syndrome)

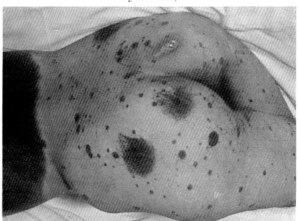

Fig. 299. Melanophakomatosis ("mélanoblastose neurocutanée")

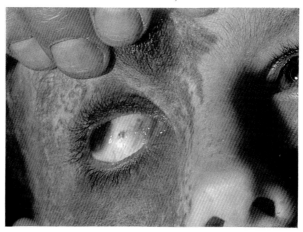

Fig. 300. Nevus Ota

Fibromas

Soft fibromas are solitary or multiple tumors, usually of hazelnut size on a broad base. Small, pedunculated, filiform fibromas, developing chiefly on the neck or near the nostrils, are seen in adults.

The chief representatives of the hard fibromas are dermatofibromas (ARNING-LEWANDOWSKY) and dermatofibroma lenticulare (SCHREUS), as well as the "nodular subepidermal fibrosis" (MICHELSON). They are pea-sized, round or oval, firm nodes, usually skin-colored but turning brownish if they have been present for a long time. They represent either genuine new formations of cells or the end stage of a granulating inflammation following some trivial trauma such as scratching or an insect bite. Their favorite site is the lower extremities. Dermatofibromas and histiocytomas do not represent different developmental phases but processes that are different from the beginning, independent of the duration. They preponderantly appear in adult females on the lower half of the body.

As in the giant cell tumors of the tendons there are multiple reticulohistiocytomas in lipoid dermatoarthritis. Here again the adult is chiefly affected. The nevoxanthoendothelioma, however, occurs in infants and small children. It has been discussed in connection with the storage diseases. Connective tissue nevi are also present in early childhood. Some of them are associated with osteopoikilosis (BUSCHKE-OLLENDORFF-CURTH). Others were already mentioned as being shagreen-like nevi located in the lumbosacral area and occurring in Morbus Bourneville-Pringle, a phakomatosis.

Keloids

In 1810 ALIBERT gave this name to sharply circumscribed, firm, pink to brownish-red, ovoid or plaque-like elevated tumors, which extend laterally like claws of lobsters and have a finely wrinkled and telangiectatic surface. They affect children and adolescents in particular, occurring mainly in the female sex. In the so-called *spontaneous keloid*, located typically over the sternum, there is not infrequently an associated folliculitis sclerotisans. In contrast, with *scar-keloids* (for example, after vaccination, skin transplantation, and burns), the rapidly growing *hypertrophic scars* remain limited to the original wound area. Familial, racial, and endocrine (thyroid, hypercalcemia) disorders as well as metabolic disturbances (porphyria) are considered causative factors in the etiology of keloids.

Lipomas

Lipomas represent characteristic soft elastic lobules or cutaneous or subcutaneous tumors. They occur on the skin as circumscribed solitary lesions (almost completely limited to adults), or multiple lesions, which appear in crops in young men. A slowly growing fatty tumor,

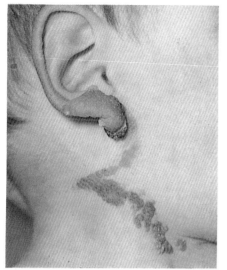

Fig. 301. Systematized verrucous nevus

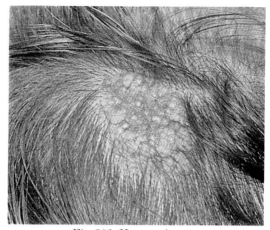

Fig. 302. Nevus sebaceus

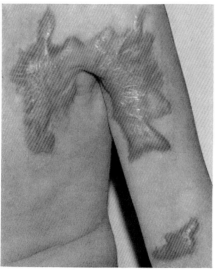

Fig. 303. Keloid

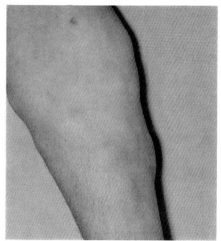

Fig. 304. Lipomas

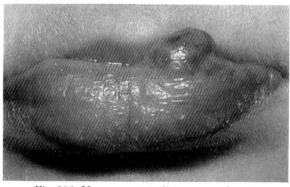

Fig. 306. Mucous cyst (salivary granuloma)

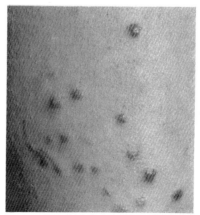

Fig. 305. Leiomyomas

which reaches the size of an apple and is located on the neck, shoulders, or axilla, is suggestive of a brown lipoma (hibernoma).

Leiomyomas

Similar to lipomas, leiomyomas occur sometimes as single but more frequently as multiple lesions. They arise on the skin from the muscles of the arrectores pilorum, those of the blood vessels, or the tunica dartos. The diagnosis is evident when characteristic sensitivity to pain is noted, such as in eccrine spiradenomas or glomus tumors. Touch, cold, caffeine, or coca-cola may cause painful muscle contractions. The lesions are usually multiple, aggregated, chiefly subcutaneous, pinhead- to pea-sized, firm, and hemispherical.

Cysts

These nodular, firmly elastic or fluctuating tumors arise either from retention of secretory material of the cutaneous glands or as genuine neoplasms from dispersed epidermal particles, as epidermoid or dermoid cysts. Familial cases of sebaceous cysts or steatomas (for example, "*atheromas*" on the scalp) occur as early as at prepuberty on the trunk or the scrotum.

Milia are chiefly found in groups on the upper two-thirds of the face. They represent pinhead-sized hard nodules filled with farina-like material. Secondary milia develop after burns or bullous cutaneous processes such as epidermolysis bullosa or porphyria cutanea tarda.

Mucous membrane cysts represent firmly elastic pea-sized elevated oral lesions. They are frequently located near the midline of the lower lip. Histologically, they represent a *mucoid granuloma*.

Hemangiomas

Hemangiomas, if one also considers their location in inner organs such as the liver, are common tumors in man. They represent either hyperplasias or hamartias. In children hemangiomas comprise 80 per cent of all tumors. This also indicates their dependency on early age. They are not infrequently associated with developmental anomalies in other tissues. Hemangiomas, especially the capillary hemangiomas, have a tendency to spontaneous regression, a unique biologic quality, as pointed out by Virchow. *Nevi flammei* are at present classified with the *nevi telangiectatici* or telangiectasis. SCHNYDER draws a sharp line between *medial-symmetric* (main example: Unna's nevus of the nape) and *lateral telangiectatic*

176

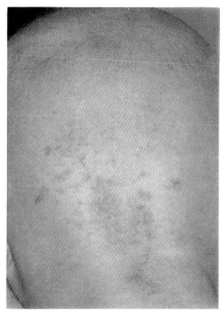

Fig. 307. Nevus flammeus of back of neck
("stork bite")

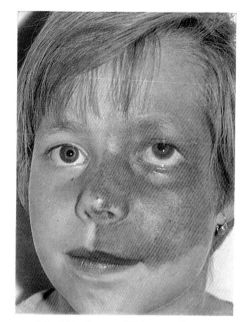

Fig. 308. Sturge-Weber syndrome

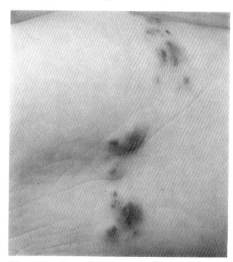

Fig. 310. Ramification of phlebectasia of
the sole

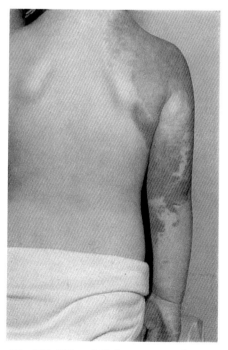

Fig. 309. Klippel-Trénaunay syndrome

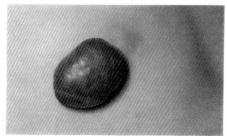

Fig. 311. Angioma cavernosum of the
breast

nevi flammei. These plain angiomas are usually present at birth. They may later show nodular transformation. They may have a segmentary distribution on the trunk. On the face they often involve the eye and oral mucosa. Occasionally they are associated with dilatations of the lymph vessels. Their functional character, evident in the beginning, is discernible in their various colors, for example, under thermic influences, when the child is crying, and during sleep.

Sturge-Weber syndrome

Associated manifestations of the nevus flammeus are the Sturge-Weber syndrome ("angiome trigéminé"), of especially the second but also the third trigeminal branch, including glaucoma, Jackson's epilepsy, or hemiparesis. This picture is considered by some authors to belong to the phakomatoses. This angiomatosis of the skin, deep ocular membranes, and the leptomeninges is probably transmitted as an irregular dominant characteristic.

Klippel-Trénaunay and Parkes-Weber syndrome

These telangiectatic nevi may be present in metameric distribution, but are in any case widely distributed, systematized, and associated with hypertrophy of connective tissue and bones. Widespread varicosities, representing rather phleb(arterio)ectases with a systolic-diastolic, practically continuous bruit over arteriovenous connections, do not occur in every case. Isolated, they develop chiefly in the first years of life, in the area of the radial or ulnar arteries. Besides functional impairment there are pigmentary disturbances, color differences, atrophies, and osseous changes, as well as protruding vascular convolutions in these areas. In a related disorder, angioma racemosum, characterized by its grape-like aspect, arterio-venous shunts, may become a dangerous load for the right side of the heart.

Papular, branching telangiectases, such as the spider-like *nevi aranei*, are observed in adults, chiefly in the presence of liver cirrhosis, in persons deficient in protein food intake, pregnant women or hyperthyroid patients. In children they present only as solitary lesions over the zygomatic bone, infrapalpebrally, or on the nose. They show a tendency to peri-pubertal involution.

Louis-Bar syndrome

This *cerebello-oculo-cutaneous telangiectatic syndrome* was observed for the first time in 1941. It is present in infants showing cerebellar ataxia with subsequent restrictions in standing and walking. Disturbed speech, dilatations of the terminal blood vessels, predominantly on the face and conjunctivae, lentigines on the trunk, prematurely white hair, sinus or bronchial infections and dystrophic retardation of growth become evident not later than in the fourth year of life. Presence of the disorder reduces life expectancy. SCHNYDER found recessive inheritance; others saw chromosomal translocations.

True vascular tumors in the infant are usually seen after the first three months and more frequently in girls than boys. These strawberry-shaped *cavernous hemangiomas* are apparently not dependent on hereditary factors. According to the structure of their surface, the hemangiomas are planotuberous or tuberonodose. Common locations are the trunk and head, and also the wrists and genitals.

178

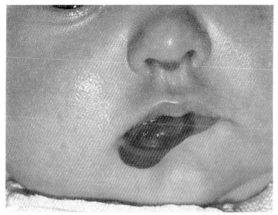

Fig. 312. Angioma cavernosum of the lip

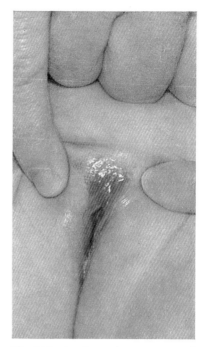

Fig. 314. Angioma cavernosum of the genitals

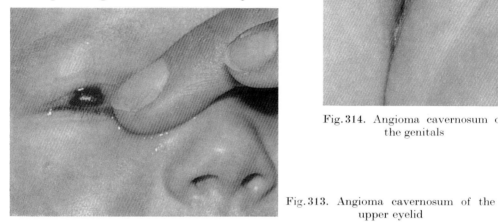

Fig. 313. Angioma cavernosum of the upper eyelid

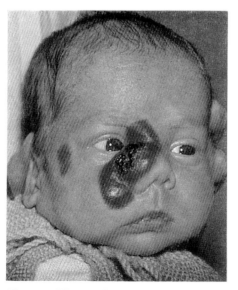

Fig. 315. Ulcerated angioma cavernosum

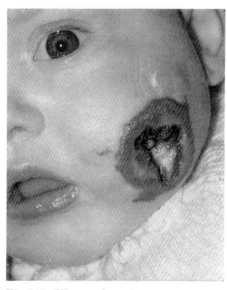

Fig. 316. Ulcerated angioma cavernosum

179

DARIER called attention to multiple progressive angiomas in children or adolescents. These tumors chiefly occur subcutaneously, and the compressible nodules have a faint blue transparence. In 1958 BEAN described multiple congenital hemangiomas, which he called the *"blue rubber-bleb nevus,"* especially of the gastrointestinal tract but also of the skin. The danger of this viscerocutaneous hemangiomatosis lies in the possibility of massive gastro-intestinal hemorrhages (hematemesis or melena) or in slow bleeding, which may lead to secondary (iron deficiency) anemia. The *Maffucci syndrome* (1881) is also characterized by multiple angiomas, associated with asymmetric chondromatosis and malformation of the limbs. The hemangiomas are accompanied by pain and increased secretion of sweat (KORTING and BREHM: hydroangioma cutis). In 1889 KAST and VON RECKLINGHAUSEN called attention to the association with pigmentary disturbances.

The *Kasabach-Merritt syndrome* (1940) presents a combination of giant hemangiomas (also in visceral location) and thrombocytopenic purpura. In some observations there was also a defibrination syndrome.

Glomus tumors

MASSON'S (1923) glomus tumor represents one of the few painful (similar to some neurinomas, leiomyomas, and eccrine spiradenomas) skin tumors and partly represents a neuromyoarterial angioma. As single lesions (on the acra or tips of the fingers) they may occur as late as in adulthood, but multiple and less painful systematized manifestations can occasionally be observed in children.

Pyogenic granuloma (Granuloma telangiectaticum benignum)

A pyogenic granuloma sits on a wide base and is a dark, fleshy-red, mostly small pedunculated formation, which reaches a certain size and remains stationary without a tendency to involution. Favorite sites are the lips or other parts of the face, and the hands. The lesions are usually solitary. The tumor corresponding to a vascular granuloma is really an eruptive angioma whose development and growth are caused by trauma and secondary infection. Neither sex is particularly favored. A pyogenic granuloma can appear at any age, although it is without a doubt most common in children.

Lymphangioma

Tumors of the lymphatic vessels appear as 1. *lymphangioma simplex* (small, frog spawn-like, transparent vesicles which, if punctured, exude a milky, lymphatic fluid, which may show admixtures of blood (hemolymphangioma); 2. *lymphangioma cavernosum* (as soft as a pillow filled with water, and covered either by normal skin or bluish-red transparent "tumors," on lips, tongue, or genitals); and finally 3. *lymphangioma cysticum* (chiefly in submaxillary location). Half the lymphangiomas, which in contrast to the angiomas rarely regress spontaneously, are evident shortly after birth. The others appear in early childhood, until about the fourteenth year of life. Lymphangiomas do not favor one sex. They are located primarily on the head or neck.

180

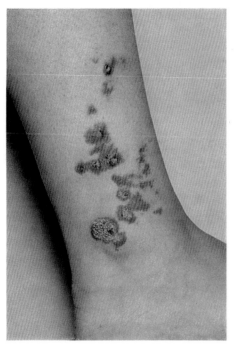

Fig. 317. Angiokeratoma (Mibelli)

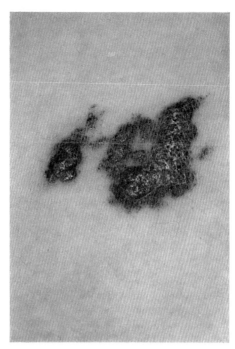

Fig. 318. Angiokeratoma (Mibelli)

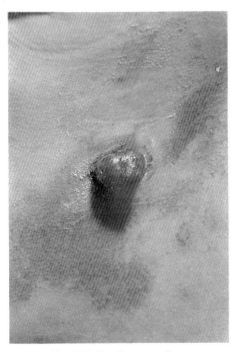

Fig. 319. Benign granuloma
teleangiectaticum

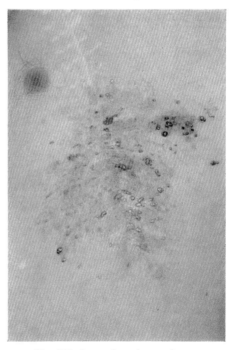

Fig. 320. Lymphangioma circum-
scriptum cysticum

181

24. Malignant Tumors of the Skin and Pigmented Tumors

Rare malignant tumors

Prenatal malignant tumors are extremely rare. These tumors are caused by diaplacental transmission of a tumor (melanoma!) of the mother or they represent primary tumors of the fetus (for example, neuroblastoma of the suprarenal glands). Among the tumors of childhood, *sarcomatous tumors* predominate. Because of their wild growth they progress rapidly and are often fatal. Of further importance in childhood, if leukemia is left out of this discussion, are tumors of the central nervous system, and mediastinal and renal tumors. The typical malignant neoplasia of the skin, the squamous cell cancer or *carcinoma spinocellulare*, as well as the *precanceroses of the skin* (according to the concept of DUBREUILH, 1896), are quite rare, most probably because of the below-threshold range of internal and external stimuli (light, cancerogenic factors, or others) and the short biometamorphosis of childhood. An exception is the autosomal recessive *xeroderma pigmentosum*, which can be compared to prematurely senile skin, predisposing the skin to epitheliomas, sarcomas, and occasionally to melanomas or neurogenic tumors as well. The rapidly developing pseudocanceroses, such as the keratoacanthoma, which shows a peak occurrence between the fiftieth and sixtieth years, are equally rare in children. Basal cell epithelioma, however, representing a locally destructive fibroepithelioma, which is dependent on the stroma, is sometimes observed in children. It may appear in nodular, nodulo-ulcerative, superficially scarring, pigmented, or cystic form. Multicentric epitheliomas on the trunk, caused by doses of arsenic given over a long period of time before manifestation, are not to be expected in children. Although basal cell epitheliomas show a peak between the fifth and seventh decades, and the atrophic skin of old age seems to be a predisposing factor, cases of epitheliomas in children have nonetheless been reported, especially in girls. The relatively common occurrence of *multiple basal cell nevi* in early childhood should be mentioned. This disorder is inherited in an autosomal dominant manner with low penetrance, whereas the common basal cell epitheliomas only exceptionally appear in several members of a family. The multiple nevi appear as discrete, up to lentil-sized tumors, chiefly centrofacially, or on the neck and the upper part of the trunk. Only rarely do they occur as nodules in linear segmentary distribution. In the beginning they are suggestive of soft nevi or neurofibromas. The *basal cell nevus syndrome* described by GORLIN and GOLTZ (1960) – already mentioned in connection with the phakomatoses – shows a characteristic syntropy with maxillary cysts and skeletal anomalies (bifurcation and fusion of ribs), and occasionally agenesis of the corpus callosum in the brain as well.

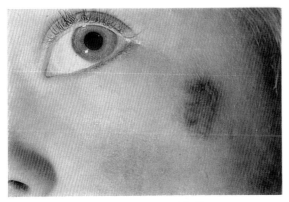

Fig. 321. Basal cell epithelioma

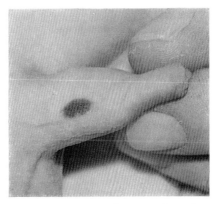

Fig. 322. Nevus cell nevus (dermal)

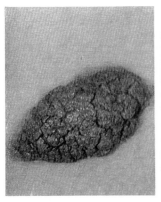

Fig. 323. Papillary nevus
cell nevus

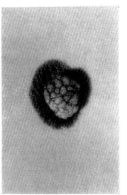

Fig. 324. Mulberry-
shaped nevus cell
nevus

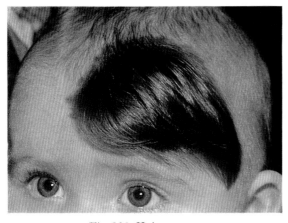

Fig. 326. Hairy nevus

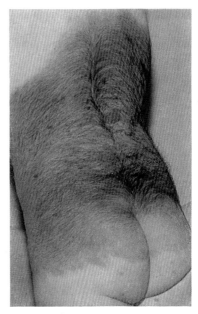

Fig. 325. Hairy nevus
(bathing trunk nevus)

Nevus cell nevi (Melanocytic nevi)

The nevus cell nevus, formerly named "pigmented nevus," is a dysontogenetic tumor on the order of highly differentiated, surprisingly evolutional and involutional, hamartomas. Most people have, after their twentieth year of life, about 20 such nevus cell nevi. On the other hand, they are rarely seen in people over the age of 90. Histologically, one differentiates nevi according to their location within the layers of the skin: 1. junction nevi, almost only in childhood, 2. compound nevi, chiefly only until puberty, and finally 3. intradermal nevus cell nevi, almost completely limited to adults. A good example of the latter is the papillary and hairy nevus cell nevus, of which the extreme expression is the classic bathing-suit nevus.

Melanoma

This tumor, which for man is malignant, arises either from a degenerating nevus cell nevus (ratio 1 in 1,000,000) on normal skin, or in older people from a "spot of old age" (*melanosis circumscripta praeblastomatosa* (Dubreuilh). The median age in 160 of our own cases of melanoma was about fifty years. According to various statistics, 1 to 2.7 per cent of all malignant melanomas occur in children.

Danger signs of transition from a pigmented nevus to a melanoma are itching or a burning sensation, an increase in size of the lesion, increasing pigmentation, either homogenously of the entire lesion or parts of the lesion, edema, oozing, bleeding, or ulceration. A red halo or small lymphatic satellites in the neighborhood are early signs of spread.

Juvenile melanoma

This special type of compound nevus was described by Sophie Spitz in 1948. A better name, which at the same time differentiates the tumor from malignant melanoma, is "spindle cell nevus" (Gertler). The nevus represents a pinhead to lentil-sized, cone-like, brownish-red or red nodule, sometimes similar to a small lesion of lupus vulgaris. Under glass pressure the nevus appears homogeneously light-brown or slate-gray. It occurs chiefly on the faces of children, between the third and thirteenth years of life. The surface of the lesion is usually smooth. In contrast to malignant melanoma, pruritus, oozing, erosions or other changes are absent. The lesion is always benign and is not a familial disorder. It is advisable to excise the lesion before puberty and to check the diagnosis histologically.

Blue nevus (Nevus caeruleus), Mongolian spot

The blue nevus, described by Jadassohn and Tièche, is usually a solitary, rice corn- to lentil-sized semispherical, dark blue tumor which usually remains benign. It is slightly

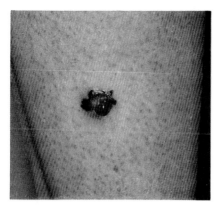

Fig. 327. Malignant melanoma

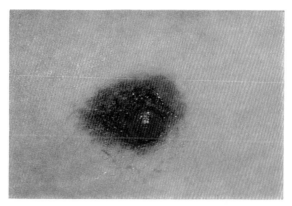

Fig. 328. Malignant melanoma

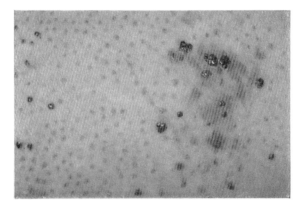

Fig. 329. Satellite melanoma – metastases located on
lichen pilaris

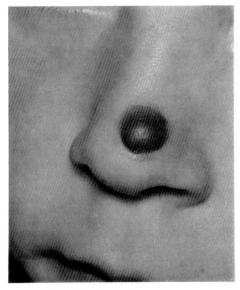

Fig. 330. Juvenile melanoma

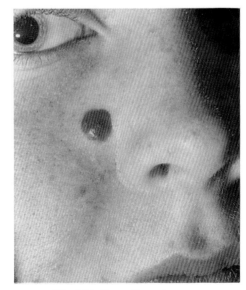

Fig. 331. Juvenile melanoma

185

lighter in the center because, in contrast to a melanoma, the follicle is spared. It consists of a three-dimensional heaping of spindle-shaped melanocytes.

Important in childhood is the "atavistic" diffuse mesodermal pigmentation of the so-called mongolian spot, which can be found over extensive areas of the sacral and coccygeal areas or the buttocks. It is usually present at birth and later regresses, around the fifth to seventh years.

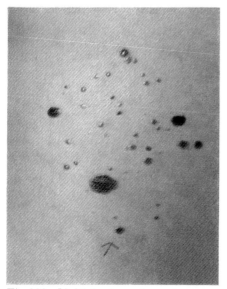

Fig. 332. Multiple juvenile melanomas

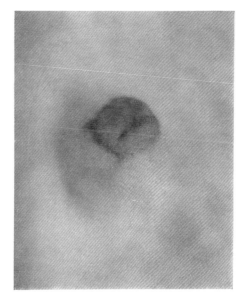

Fig. 333. Nevus caeruleus
(blue nevus of Jadassohn)

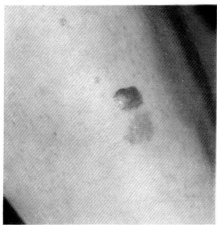

Fig. 334. Nevus caeruleus and nevus cell
nevus adjacent to each other

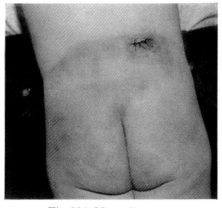

Fig. 336. Mongolian spot

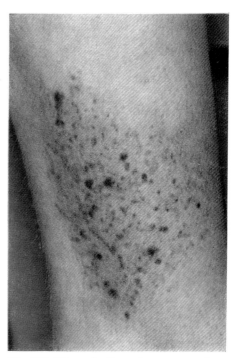

Fig. 335. Dissemination of nevus caeruleus
and multiple nevus cell nevi

25. Leukemias, Lymphomas, and Reticuloendothelioses

Leukemias

These disorders are regarded today as uncontrolled, irreversible, progressive proliferations of elements of one of the three blood cell lines. They are either genuine tumors or hyperplasias, or may represent the result of virus infections. In childhood we deal chiefly with the acute, rapidly developing cutaneous picture of lymphadenosis (BISIADECKI, 1876) (lymphatic leukemia) or of myelosis (BRUUSGARD, 1911) (myelogenous leukemia). Chronic lymphatic leukemia, in contrast, occurs at an advanced age and shows the highest degree of cutaneous involvement of all the leukemias, that is, in about one-third of the patients. Basically, 90 per cent of all accompanying cutaneous manifestations, which cannot always be classified histologically, are nonspecific (PINKUS). These are the leukemids (AUDRY). The *acute leukemias with immature cells* frequently begin, as do the other forms, with uncharacteristic (pallor, fever, arthritis) or typical (anemia, lessened resistance to infection) signs; but here a severe *hemorrhagic diathesis as a main sign is noteworthy*. There are crops of ecchymoses, chiefly in the sacral area, and hemorrhages, such as are seen in generalized septic conditions. In the oral cavity they simulate severe scurvy. Also suspect are stubborn nosebleeds or hemorrhages from the gastrointestinal tract. Hematuria, however, is rare.

In *monocytic leukemia*, dark, fetid, necrotic, ulcerative lesions of the gums, occasionally following dental treatment, or similar changes on the palatal arch or the tonsils are predominant in 80 per cent of all patients.

In a few instances manifestations have been seen in children shortly after birth (so-called congenital cutaneous leukemia). They were either polymorphic, exanthematous, especially maculopapular or rubelliform eruptions which, however, could also simulate erythema annulare, erythema multiforme, or tumorous infiltrations. Urticarial lesions predominate among the uncharacteristic manifestations, but pruriginous reactions (prurigo lymphatica) following a chronic course are also seen. In contrast to the polymorphic exanthems of childhood, chronic lymphatic leukemia, favoring males of advanced ages and hardly ever occurring in adolescents, shows the complete picture of an "acrodermatosis," a leonine face with blue-red, lupoid, plaque-like or tuberous infiltrations, and a telangiectatic surface. Generalized herpes zoster and priapism are associated signs.

Reticuloendothelioses

Letterer-Siwe and Hand-Schüller-Christian Disease

In 1924 LETTERER observed a disorder related to leukemias or aleukemias showing pro-liferation of the reticuloendothelial system. In subsequent years the concept of reticulo-endothelioses was used for all disorders of the reticulohistiocytic system. These disorders begin multicentrically and are associated with an increase in reticulogenic elements of the cells. They represent new growths of the reticulohistiocytary system or the third line of blood cells, having the character of autonomous systemic neoplasias. Occasionally the skin is a site of such reticuloendothelioses.

Not belonging to reticulosis cutis in the narrow neoplastic sense are the so-called orthoplastic and metaplastic reticuloendothelioses, or – if one considers possible spontaneous regression or reversibility – the certain reactive reticulum cell increases, which are closely associated with chronic inflammation. A better classification for these is *reticular hyperplasia* (GOTTRON), or reticulocytosis (LENNERT and ELSCHNER). The malignant, chiefly sarcomatous, retothelial tumors and the *lipid storage disorders* should not be classified with the reticuloendothelioses. Such disorders are caused by a disturbed metabolism of the reticulum cells with subsequent accumula-tion of lipids in the cells, but they are not based on a primary neoplasia of reticulum cell elements.

The cytologically monomorphic and histologically initial cutaneous reticuloendothelioses (in a limited sense), located at the skin appendages, are large tuberous, plaque-like, small tuberous-exanthematous and primary erythrodermatous variants, systemically involve the viscera, including the lymph nodes, relatively late (before death), and show an abundance of circulating monocytes. To this type belong characteristic pictures: the so-called *reticulo-sarcomatosis cutis* (GOTTRON), which is rapidly destructive like the multiple autochthonous paramyeloblast leukemias, and the Sézary syndrome with erythroderma and leukemia of the blood.

Even in earliest childhood there are reticuloendothelioses with cutaneous manifestations. They also differ clinically and histologically from Letterer-Siwe disease. This disorder, however, is the prevalent form of reticuloendotheliosis in childhood. This *reticuloendotheliosis of the infant*, the disorder which led to LETTERER's concept of reticuloendotheliosis, the lipoid granulomatosis (Hand-Schüller-Christian type) and *eosinophilic granuloma* are the same disease, occasionally called *histiocytosis* X (LICHTENSTEIN, 1953). These three types progress differently: reticuloendotheliosis of the infant represents an accelerated variant associated with fever, anemia, and hepatosplenomegaly, but only sparse eosinophilia in the cutaneous manifestations; Hand-Schüller-Christian disease shows xanthomatous infiltrations. The initial finding of all three syndromes, however, is the reticuloendotheliosis.

Letterer-Siwe disease, which exclusively affects children up to the second year of life, may take a stormy, septic course. The eruption is characterized by dry, occasionally icteric skin, seborrheic-like erythema, and up to rice kernel-sized, squamous, crusted papules, as in Darier's disease. There is also purpura, even on the palmoplantar surfaces. The bones, chiefly the mastoid, are affected. Numerous patients suffer from running ears with character-istic granulation tissue in the external ear canal. A specific gingivitis is not uncommon.

190

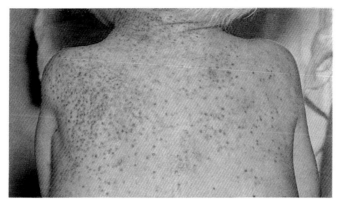

Fig. 337. Letterer-Siwe disease (Hand-Schüller-Christian disease in a child)

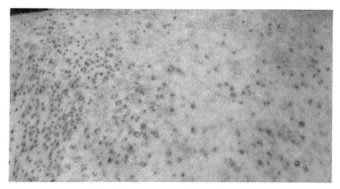

Fig. 338. Letterer-Siwe disease

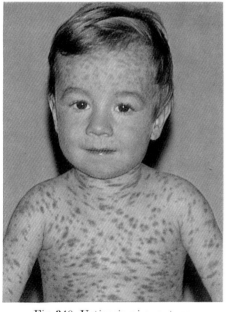

Fig. 340. Urticaria pigmentosa

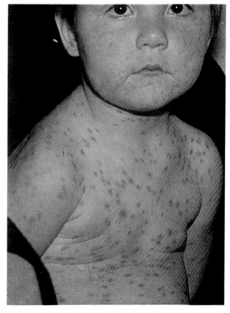

Fig. 341. Urticaria pigmentosa

Hand-Schüller-Christian disease begins slowly in children aged 3 to 5 years. If it starts later – around the sixteenth year of life – its prognosis is more favorable. About one-third of the patients has cutaneous signs similar to those in reticuloendotheliosis of infants. Later, disseminated xanthomas varying from papules to tubers are observed on dry, pale or brownish skin (hoarseness is caused by xanthomas on the vocal cords). Occasionally, characteristic swellings of the scalp appear. These are caused by osteolytic lesions of the skull. Other main signs are exophthalmos and diabetes insipidus. Patients complain of headaches or pain in the legs.

Eosinophilic granuloma (FINZI, 1929; LICHTENSTEIN and JAFFÉ, 1940) shows few signs. It looks like Hand-Schüller-Christian disease, with seborrhea-like erythemas and papules as in Darier's disease. The characteristic lesions are large, eroded or granulomatous vegetating lesions which occur mostly in the axillae or the genitoanal region.

Urticaria pigmentosa

Urticaria pigmentosa was named by SANGSTER in 1878. The disease was originally observed by the ophthalmologist NETTLESHIP in 1869 in a two-year-old child, the initial signs having appeared in the third month of life. This disease is now considered to be a mast cell reticuloendotheliosis. Mast cell reticuloendotheliosis (SÉZARY, 1952), or the less apt *mastocytosis* (SÉZARY, 1936), which, incidentally, can occur without cutaneous manifestations, should be differentiated from basophilic or mast cell leukemia. Almost limited to adults, it presents as a systemic neoplastic proliferation of more immature mast cells than the classic form of urticaria pigmentosa, which is limited to the skin, is benign, and is reversible. LENNERT and SCHUBERT contend that cytologic differentiation can be made by examination with a buffered toluidine-blue pH chain; GRÜNEBERG, however, does not concur. Nevertheless, it must be admitted that even in classic urticaria pigmentosa mast cell infiltrates can occur in the sternal bone marrow or other parts of the osseous system (SAGHER), as well as in the liver, spleen, and gastrointestinal tract, where it may be associated with diarrhea, colic, and vomiting. Osseous changes are chiefly osteosclerotic and less frequently osteoporotic or mixed. Other findings are periosteal formations, compacta islands, increased trabeculae, cysts, and a narrowing of the marrow-containing cavities.

In the reversible reticular hyperplasia of the mast cell type, lesions occur as a few, single, large tumorous manifestations (solitary mastocytoma), in early infancy (75 per cent). In young adults they more often appear as small, densely scattered macules, leaving the face, palms, soles, and oral cavity free and involving predominantly the trunk and extremities, with light yellow, yellow-brown to brown, pinhead to coin-sized lesions. If one rubs these lesions they swell up so typically (sign of DARIER) that if this reaction fails to appear the clinical diagnosis should be verified by histologic examination.

This swelling is explained by the release of the histamine (RILEY and WEST) present in the mast cell granules and discharged when the lesion is rubbed. If extensive amounts of histamine are released (for instance following rubbing after a hot bath), the circulation may be impaired. The cytoplasm of the mast cells, however, contains apparently heparin-like substances which may be responsible for the pigmentation and occasional disturbances of blood coagulability. Specific differences in serotonin in mast cells seem to be present in the various animal species.

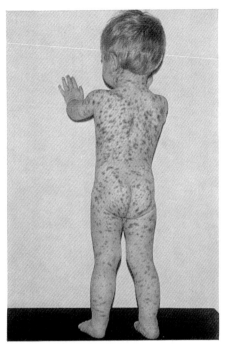

Fig. 339. Urticaria pigmentosa

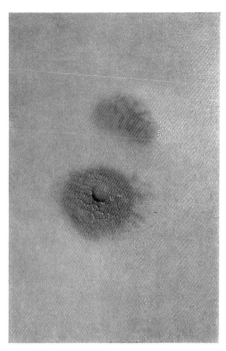

Fig. 342. Solitary mastocytoma

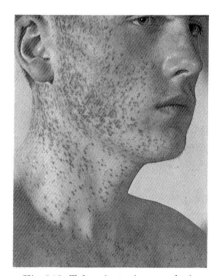

Fig. 343. Telangiectasia macularis
eruptiva perstans

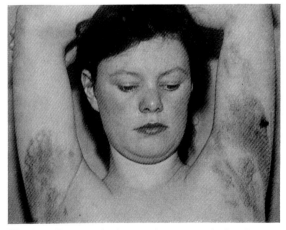

Fig. 344. Parapsoriasis en plaques, reticular hyperplasia following nitrofurantoin

Dermographia and pruritus vary from case to case and are therefore unreliable diagnostic signs. The individual lesion may, on account of its tumor-like form and yellow color, suggest xanthoma (TILBURY FOX: *urticaria pigmentosa xanthelasmoidea*). Blisters within the lesions, urticaria pigmentosa pemphigoides, occur rather infrequently. F. B. WEBER and HELLEN-SCHMIED (1930) described a telangiectatic modification with diminution of the pigment as *telangiectasia macularis eruptiva perstans*. Patients with this variant tend to develop peptic ulcers and, based on our own observations, complain of irradiating symptoms of Raynaud's disease.

Cutaneous manifestations in plasmacytoma and macroglobulinemia (multiple myelomas)

The modulation and transformation of the plasma cell in the reticuloendothelioses reaches its fullest expression in the plasma cell leukemias, *plasmocytoma* or *multiple myeloma* (KAHLER, 1889). Corresponding cellular findings (plasmocytes in the bone marrow and the peripheral blood streamly) exist along with the protein-chemical evidence of the paraproteinemia (with extremely high ESR and high alpha, beta, or gamma values with small peaks on electrophoresis; evidence of paraproteins by ultracentrifugation of the entire serum; and urinary paraproteins: Bence-Jones proteins, "paraproteinemic nephrosis"). Osseous changes (sharply limited light zones or diffuse osteoporosis) are visualized radiologically. Specific *cutaneous changes* are chiefly tumorous and are reminiscent of tumors of mycosis fungoides or reticuloendothelial sarcomas. Nontumorous cutaneous changes are all nonspecific and, because of their polymorphism, nondiagnostic. However, paramyloidal changes (or systemic amyloidosis), frequently associated with the plasmacytoma, may show characteristic changes similar to scleroderma amyloidosum (GOTTRON), including macroglossia (LUBARSCH).

Moderate *macroglobulinemia* may appear during the first year of life in the serum of healthy children and symptomatically in the complex bleeding tendency of syphilitic infants. In later life, especially in old age, symptomatic macroglobulinemias accompany systemic disorders (reticuloendothelioses, leukemias, plasmocytomas, or other neoplastic diseases). The cutaneous lesions of "essential" Waldenström's disease, accompanied by hepatosplenomegaly and enlarged lymph nodes, are secondary and uncharacteristic, especially when associated with cryoglobulinemia. They appear as purpura, Raynaud's syndrome, ulcerative lesions of the acra, or acrodermatitis chronica atrophicans, and they are accompanied by bleeding from the nose and oral cavity. The tumorous, cutaneous type of Waldenström's disease, which GOTTRON, KORTING, and NIKOLOWSKI described for the first time in 1960, has been observed several times since.

Systemic reticulogranulomatoses

Lymphogranulomatosis of the skin (Paltauf-Sternberg disease or Hodgkin's disease)

Individuals of every age group may suffer from reticulogranulomatosis. Children and very old people, however, are not often affected. The peak incidence occurs between the second and fourth decades, and the male sex is slightly favored. The etiology of the disorder is not clearly understood. The question of whether we are dealing with an inflammation (granuloma) or a neoplasia induced by a virus with questionable possibilities of development into a genuine sarcoma or a tumor of a rather benign character (paragranuloma, JACKSON and PARKER) is still controversial. The classification of clinical signs is easier; cutaneous-lympho-nodular, cervical, or cervico-axillary mediastinal-plurinodular subtypes have been observed. Initial abdominal manifestations may not be correctly diagnosed for a long time.

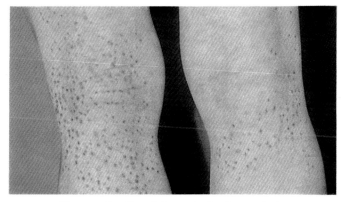

Fig. 345. Small nodular reticular hyperplasia

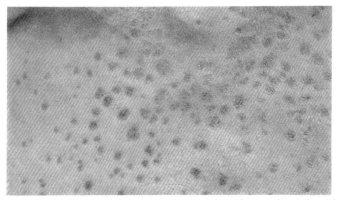

Fig. 346. Reticular hyperplasia (similar to diffuse leukemia of the skin)

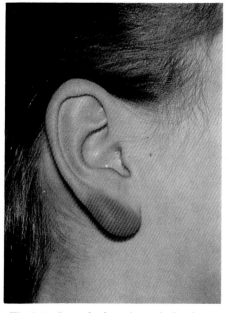

Fig. 347. Lymphadenosis cutis benigna
(lymphocytoma)

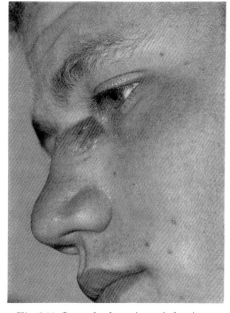

Fig. 348. Lymphadenosis cutis benigna

Signs and symptoms are periodic high fever (PEL-EBSTEIN), leukopenia, acute dysprotein-emia, diazo reaction in the urine, and pain at the site of the disease after the ingestion of alcohol. In this "malignant granuloma" there are either specific infiltrations, nonspecific cutaneous manifestations (S. GROSZ, 1906), or a mixture of both. Characteristic are further paroxysms of violent pruritus, other symptoms, and urticarial and pruriginous eruptions. Lichenified, eczematoid lesions, erythroderma, and poikiloderma are seen less frequently. Still less often observed are eruptions resembling erythema multiforme, nodosum, or hemorrhagicum. The specific cutaneous changes are preponderantly tumor-like papular or plaque-like infiltrations which often break down, forming long lasting "ulcera lympho-granulomatosa" (ARZT and RANDAK). These may become extensive. Lymphogranulomatosis which has extended into the skin by infiltration of contiguous specific granulomatous tissue in contiguity from other organs is not unusual.

Mycosis fungoides (granuloma fungoides)

Mycosis fungoides affects adults in the fourth to sixth decades, without preference of sex. Onset of the disorder before the twentieth year of life is unusual.

The classic type (D'ALIBERT-BAZIN) is progressive. Characteristics of the initial stage are variable and may include urticaria, prurigo, eczema, or parapsoriasis-like pruritic erythema with a tendency to lichenification or horny plugs. After a period of years the second stage of mycotic infiltration is seen; the final stage of mycotic tumors follows. In exceptional cases of mycosis fungoides the initial eruption is an erythroderma (type HALLOPEAU-BESNIER or LEREDDE), whereas "mycose d'emblée" (VIDAL-BROCQ) without a "premycotic" phase, usually represents a reticuloendotheliomatous sarcoma. In contrast to Hodgkin's disease, pruritus or other sensations are no certain diagnostic criteria.

Reticular hyperplasias of the skin

Histologically characteristic of this group is the proliferation of lymphoreticular cells forming granulomas. The disorder may vary from case to case, with more lymphatic or reticuloendothelial features, a preponderance of plasma cells, or greater follicular involvement. The chief representative of this group of reversible hyperplasias (and other reticular cutaneous hyperplasias which constitute responses to irritations or stimuli) is lymphadenosis benigna cutis.

Lymphadenosis benigna cutis (Lymphocytoma)

Under the name of lymphadenosis benigna cutis, BÄFVERSTEDT grouped the following disorders: SPIEGLER-FENDT's (1894 and 1900) sarcoid and lymphocytoma (BIBERSTEIN, 1923), which had been described earlier (1921) by MARIE KAUFMANN-WOLF as "benign lymphocytic neoplasia of the scrotal skin of the child." Single or multiple lesions develop relatively slowly in the cutis or subcutis. The lesions may develop in a disseminated or generalized fashion. Gray-brown, plaque-like or flat, atrophic, and tuberous or miliary, the lesions rarely ulcerate. They cause little discomfort and tend to regress spontaneously. The lesions may simulate lupus vulgaris nodules, but a probe will not sink in. Limited types favor the face. Characteristic in children are light or dusky red-blue infiltrations of the ear lobe, less frequently of the scrotum or the areola. Sometimes one finds the development of such solitary lymphocytomas secondary to a tick bite, as in erythema migrans and acrodermatitis chronica atrophicans. The successful experimental transmission of lymphocytoma tissue from a patient to a healthy individual (PASCHOUD, 1957) also speaks in favor of infectious disease, at least in some cases. Much less frequent is an association with malignant processes.

Lymphadenosis benigna cutis can occur at any age. It is not at all infrequent in small children, even infants. Solitary lymphocytomas are seen primarily in children and adolescents, favoring the male sex. In older age groups mostly women are affected.

A clinical variant of such benign "lymphoplasias" (MACH) is lymphocytic infiltration (JESSNER and KANOF, 1953) with brownish-red, flat, discoid lesions, which in contrast to chronic lupus erythematosus are smooth and without follicular hyperkeratosis. They are located predominantly on the face, and may be provoked by exposure to light.

26. Diseases of the Sweat Glands

Dyshidrosis, miliaria, and chromhidrosis

Complete (anatomic) absence of sweat glands occurs only in association with other ectodermal defects (of the teeth, hair, nails; faulty development of sebaceous and mammary glands, anosmia, ozena) as a definite familial entity, chiefly in the male sex (anhidrosis hypotrichotica).

Dyshidrosis (T. Fox, 1873; Hutchinson: Cheiropomphclyx, 1876) is one of the dyshidrosiform skin reactions, with subgroups such as dyshidrosiform mycids, pyodermas, eczemas, and hematogenic-toxic exanthems. In children, especially, focal toxic influences (particularly from the tonsils) have to be considered.

Miliaria (sudamina and prickly heat) represents chiefly a sweat retention syndrome, which may manifest either superficially, like tears on the skin (Trousseau), or, according to the involvement of different layers of the skin, as miliaria crystallina, rubra, pustulosa, or profunda in moist heat (overheated infants' wards) fever, sunburn, and so forth. It is mostly of short duration.

Colored sweat *(chromhidrosis)* can be the result of a patient's occupation and is therefore a disorder of later age. Red impregnation of underwear may be caused by *trichomycosis axillaris (palmellina)* of the axillary hair.

Granulosis rubra nasi

This disorder with acneiform or rosacea-like changes in the neighborhood of the tip of the nose was described by Pringle, Luithlen, and J. Jadassohn. It may occur in several members of a family and is often associated with frost-bite, acrocyanosis and Feer's disease.

Fox-Fordyce disease

This "rare papular disease of the axillary region" was described in 1902. It also affects the nipples, the umbilicus, and the genitoperineal region. The small, pinhead-sized, flat to conical, prominent, skin-colored tumors appear in the area of the apocrine glands and are associated with severe itching. Presence of the disease before puberty is exceptional.

198

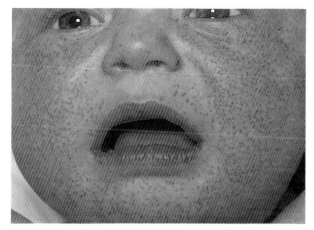

Fig. 350. Miliaria (sudamina)

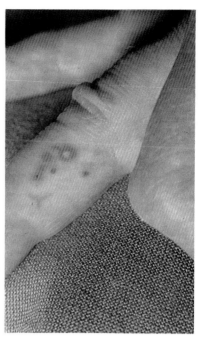

Fig. 349. Dyshidrosis

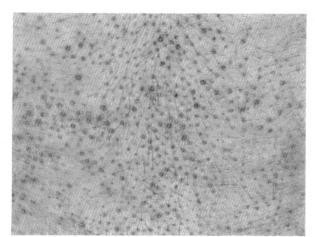

Fig. 351. Miliaria rubra

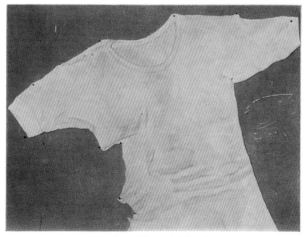

Fig. 352. Chromhidrosis

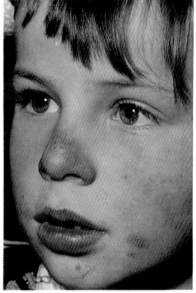

Fig. 353. Granulosis rubra nasi

27. Diseases of the Sebaceous Glands

Acne vulgaris

Acne vulgaris is characterized by the simultaneous occurrence of osteofollicular keratoses (comedones) and papulopustular infiltrations. Distribution of the lesions is limited to the face and the upper parts of the trunk. This dermatosis of peripuberty usually runs in families. It is provoked by certain foods. *Acne conglobata* (SPITZER and LANG), in contrast, is characterized by grouped or giant comedones, connecting or irregular scars, pressure atrophies, and a cutis laxa type of integument. It may be found on the buttocks, thighs, and so forth.

Occupational acne, which may occur in adolescent apprentices, is usually as monomorphic as drug induced acneiform eruption (following administration of adrenocorticotropic hormone, cortisone, testosterone, isoniazid, vitamin D, and others).

Acneiform eruptions of infants and small children (acne neonatorum and infantum) are rare. They occur exclusively on the face and favor the cheeks or the forehead, either as grouped comedones or as papulopustules ("puberty in miniature"). From the small sebaceous retention cysts, present since the second week of life with conspicuous persistence, KLOSTERMANN and NIETZKI isolated yeast (candida parapsilosis). Contact with skin creams ("edema from petrolatum" OPPENHEIM) or massive vitamin D_2 therapy may also cause acneiform eruptions.

Neurotic excoriations ("acne excoriée des jeunes filles," BROCQ, 1898) are observed chiefly on the face. They represent flat, lenticular, often thickly crusted lesions which leave many scars because of the constant manipulations of the patient.

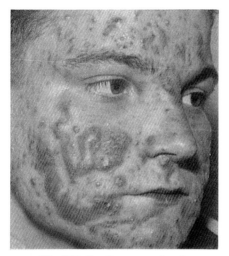

Fig. 354. Cystic acne vulgaris

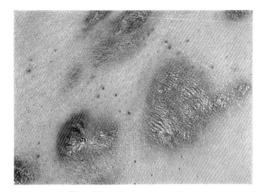

Fig. 355. Acne conglobata

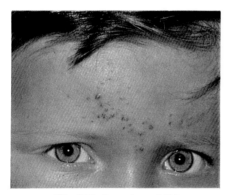

Fig. 356. Acne in a child

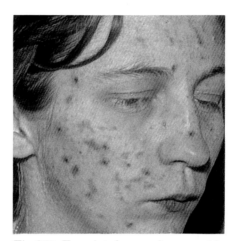

Fig. 358. Excoriated acne of young girls

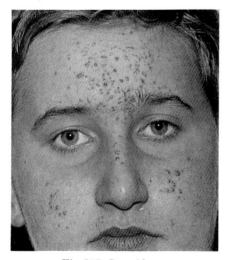

Fig. 357. Steroid acne

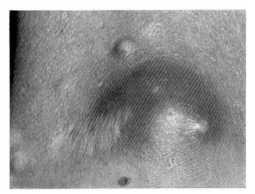

Fig. 359. Sebaceous retention cysts (so-called pseudoatheromas)

28. Diseases of the Hair

Congenital anomalies of the hair are relatively uncommon. They favor the male sex and are frequently associated with other malformations, such as hidrotic and anhidrotic ectodermal dysplasias and polydysplasias.

Monilethrix and other congenital deviations of hair growth

Aplasia pilorum moniliformis (monilethrix) is uncommon and is a dominant inherited disorder. It is associated with malformations, such as keratosis pilaris, or disturbances of nail growth (HEYDT: in almost 70 per cent of patients koilonychia, or "spoon nails," is present). The moniliform hairs, noticeable in childhood after about the first year of life, are characterized by alternate constrictions or more heavily pigmented spindle-shaped swellings. At the same time, the hair is dry and breaks off easily, especially in the occipital area. The resulting baldness is more or less complete and the scalp slowly becomes atrophic.

Hypotrichosis congenita hereditaria was described in 1925 by M. UNNA. The afflicted infant shows congenital lack of hair with retarded development of bristly, often twisted and fragile hair, gradually leading to alopecia.

Other anomalies are *pili torti*, *anulati*, and *planati*, and *kinky* or *woolly* hair. In *trichostasis spinulosa* a cluster or tuft of ten or more fine hairs grows out of a single strongly keratotic follicle.

Exogenous hair damage

Alopecia occipitalis s. decubitalis

Since infants lay on their backs most of the time, the occipital region is mechanically abused. In infancy loss of hair in this area is almost physiologic. As soon as the infant begins to sit up and the insults cease, there is restitution of hair.

Trichotillomania (Hallopeau)

"Alopécie manuelle" (BROCQ), the urge to pull out the hairs, may be observed in children and occasionally even in infants, who seem to obtain satisfaction from this action. Various parts of the scalp, predominantly the vertex but occasionally the eyelashes and eyebrows as well, are chosen sites.

Intensive, persistent traction of the hair, for example, in girls who wear a "pony-tail," may cause so-called *traction alopecia*.

Structural changes

Trichoclasis (JACKSON-SABOURAUD) occurs not only in idiopathic form but also in association with other diseases of the hair. Most of the structural changes of the hair, as in *trichonodosis* (knotted hairs), *trichoschisis* (split hairs), *trichorrhexis nodosa*, are caused by mechanical maltreatment (scratching, hot waving, brushing with hard bristles, and so forth) and are therefore observed mostly in adults.

Changes in color of the hair

In children color changes are seen in albinism, vitiligo, in hair regrowing in areas of alopecia areata, or in heterochromias (congenital hair color differences occurring in stripes, spots, or in diffuse or circumscribed areas). The changes may also constitute part of a syndrome, for example, the white, thin hair of children with kwashiorkor, or the almost transparent, thin hair of patients with phenylketonuria.

Quantitative changes (hypertrichoses)

Familial cases have been seen in which the downy lanugo hair of the infant is not replaced by the fully developed hair of the adult. Acquired *hypertrichosis lanuginosa*, however, points to malnutrition (insufficient food intake or cachexia from a tumor). If local hypertrichosis, secondary hypertrichosis, or response to external irritations are disregarded, hirsutism points to hyperpituitarism or other pituitary or diencephalic disturbances. Disorders of the ovaries such as arrhenoblastomas or polycystic ovaries (Stein-Leventhal's syndrome) may also play a role. In children, generalized hypertrichoses may follow treatment with certain drugs (cortisone, hydantoin). *Coccygeal hypertrichosis* points to a status dysraphicus. A deep posterior hairline on the nape is chiefly observed in gonadal dysgenesis (Turner's syndrome) or in Down's syndrome.

Acquired alopecias (alopecia areata)

Congenital alopecia commonly leads to follicular or cicatricial atrophy. *Acquired alopecias*, however, heal to a great extent without scars and are therefore prognostically favorable with regard to renewed hair growth. They are either circumscribed or diffuse (following infections, chiefly typhoid, secondary to syphilis, or after poisons such as arsenic, mercury, thallium, anticoagulants, or cytotoxic drugs).

The most important circumscribed hair loss in young people is *alopecia areata* (area celsi, pelade), which may begin abruptly or gradually. In over half the cases the alopecia is located over the occiput (the prognostically unfavorable "ophiasis"), and in about a quarter of cases it is located in the fronto-vertical region. If the hair of the entire scalp has fallen out because of confluence of affected areas, we speak of alopecia totalis seu maligna. Alopecia universalis may also affect the beard, chest, armpits, and genital area. In alopecia areata hairs fall out with the root. They grow back silky-soft and with little pigment. During the interval without hair the affected area acquires an ivory color through diminution of pigment and simultaneous hyperplasia of sebaceous glands (RICHTER). Very fine stippling of the nails is

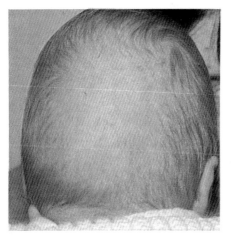

Fig. 360. Decubital alopecia

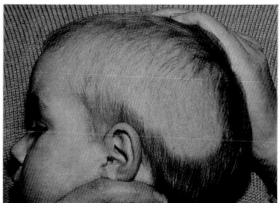

Fig. 361. Trichotillomania

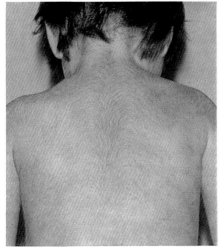

Fig. 362. Hypertrichosis lanuginosa

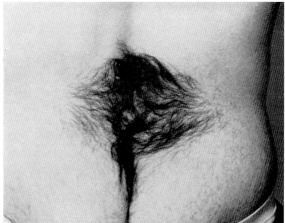

Fig. 363. Hypertrichosis sacralis associated with spina bifida occulta

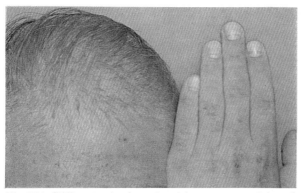

Fig. 364. Diffuse toxic alopecia with transverse striae of the nails after administration of thallium

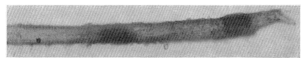

Fig. 365. Segmentary melanin clusters of the hair in alopecia caused by thallium

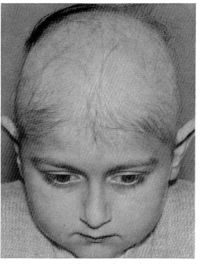

Fig. 366. Diffuse alopecia after cyclophosphamide

associated (GALEWSKY, BETTMANN, KLINGMÜLLER) in some cases of familial alopecia. If alopecia areata has begun before puberty, it has an unfavorable prognosis (frequent recurrences). Familial cases may be associated with Horner's syndrome (LANGHOF) or other defects such as mongolism (KORTING and HOLZMANN). Focal infections frequently cause hair loss. According to BRAUN-FALCO, alopecia areata is a mixed alopecia, that is, a combination of an alopecia of club hairs (telogen hairs) and a primarily dystrophic alopecia caused by an enzymatous defect in the mitotically active hair matrix.

In contrast to alopecia areata, *pseudopelade*, or alopecia atrophicans BROCQ, exhibits in young adults smooth, bald, atrophic areas, which can be compared to footprints in the snow.

Alopecia mucinosa (H. Pinkus)

Follicular papules with horny plugs (thus giving a spinulous aspect) characterize the clinical picture of this circumscribed alopecia caused by follicular and seboglandular mucinosis. It may occur in children. In adults it may point to an association with a systemic reticuloendotheliosis such as mycosis fungoides (KORTING).

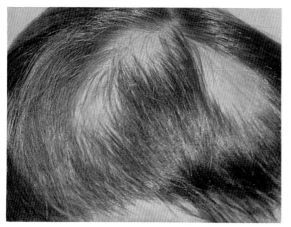

Fig. 367. Alopecia areata

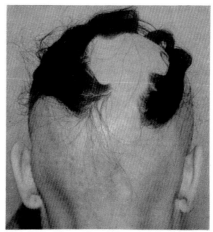

Fig. 369. Alopecia of the occipital region
(ophiasis)

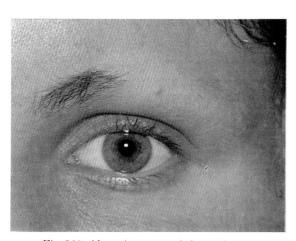

Fig. 368. Alopecia areata of the eyebrows

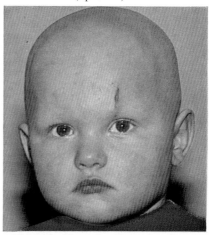

Fig. 370. Alopecia areata totalis or
maligna

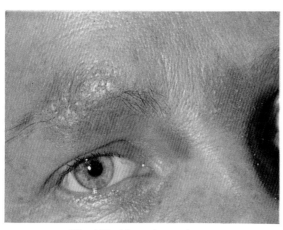

Fig. 372. Alopecia mucinosa

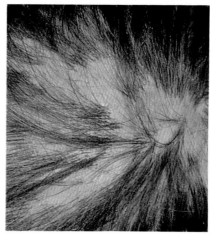

Fig. 371. Pseudopelade Brocq

207

29. Diseases of the Nails

Between the fifth and thirtieth years of life the fingernails grow an average of 0.1 mm. per day. In general, hyperemia accelerates and ischemia slows the growing process. The basic changes in clubbing of the nails consist of an increase in the volume of the soft tissue of the terminal phalanx of the digits. This condition occurs in patients with chronic pleuropulmonary and cardiovascular disorders, biliary cirrhosis, and as a sign of congenital familial disease. In *onychopathias*, changes in the form, color, and consistency of the nails occur. Congenital total or subtotal *aplasias of the nails* are associated chiefly with congenital anomalies of the fingers or hands, or with congenital dermatoses such as epidermolysis bullosa hereditaria of the dystrophic type. Color changes of the nail plate are caused by external factors or fungi. *Leukonychia*, the whitish discoloration of the nails, can have many causes. It may even occur as a congenital anomaly, or may be caused by febrile disease, pellagra, or intake of thallium. *Mee's nail band*, showing the color of the lunula, is caused by a single arsenic intoxication. The form of the nail plate is changed in *spoon nails* (BALL, R. CROCKER), or *koilonychia* (HELLER, KATZNELSON), which may be present at birth or appear in childhood. Other causes are chiefly lack of iron or vitamin B_2. Children do not show the effects of mechanical trauma or damage from alkali. Nail biting (onychophagia) causes the curved nail to become flat. This may lead to koilonychia. Transverse nail furrows (Beau's lines, 1896) indicate a harmful influence at a certain time. Infants may show this sign from changes in nutrition. The etiology of a half-moon shaped detachment *(onycholysis semilunaris partialis)* of the fingernail is unexplained. Onycholysis following exposure to light may occur in children taking demethylchlortetracycline. Pathologically increased brittleness of the nails, which is caused by increased splitting and disintegration (onychorrhexis DUBREUILH, 1896) may occur in early childhood. On the other hand, *hapalonychia*, a pathologic softening of the nail substance, is not particularly common in young people. Although *onychogryposis* (deformed overgrowth of the nail) may be present at birth, it is more often observed at older ages when there are more frequent disturbances of blood supply. In young people, acute pyogenic onychias and most *paronychias* are caused by infections arising from inadequate nail care. Staphylococci and yeast (Monilia) are the causative organisms. The latter cause subacute paronychias, chiefly in women.

208

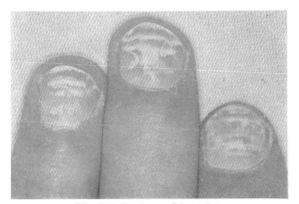

Fig. 373. Leukonychia striata

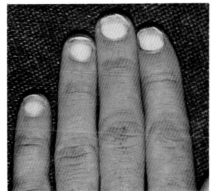

Fig. 374. Leukonychia totalis

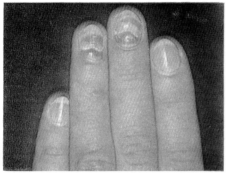

Fig. 375. Reil-Beau's lines

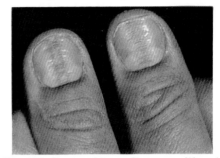

Fig. 376. Dystrophia mediana canaliformis

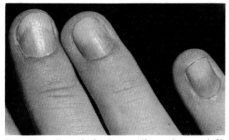

Fig. 377. Onycholysis semilunaris partialis

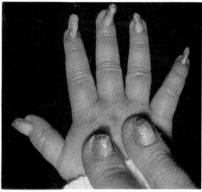

Fig. 379. Pachyonychia congenita

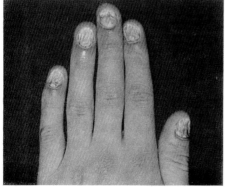

Fig. 378. Onychorrhexis (differential
diagnosis: onychomycosis)

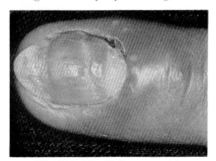

Fig. 380. Monilial paronychia

30. Diseases of the Oral Mucosa and Tongue

Heterotopic sebaceous cysts (Fordyce's disease)

Fordyce's disease occurs on the inner lips and the gums between the teeth, less frequently on the vermilion border, and occasionally on the female genitals (small labia). In newborns and infants such grouped, enlarged, heterotopic sebaceous glands are as a rule not present. Seborrhea and endogenous eczema are not associated with Fordyce's disease. Menopausal women and both sexes after puberty, however, may be affected.

Leukoplakia

Congenital leukoplakias, known by various names, occur more frequently on the buccal mucosa than on the tongue. Leukoplakias are present in Darier's disease, ichthyosis congenita, dystrophic epidermolysis bullosa hereditaria, polykeratosis congenita Touraine, and pachyonychia congenita. Other more common leukoplakias are observed at a later age.

Glossitis rhombica mediana (Brocq-Pautrier)

Medially located in the middle third of the tongue at the tuberculum impar, there may be a benign fissural anomaly, presenting a rhombic area without papillae. Less frequently an oval, sharply limited, leukoplakic verrucous change is seen. In children the anomaly is barely visible.

Lingua geographica

Lingua geographica is basically a harmless constitutional anomaly. The sharply limited exfoliations of the tongue are seldom fixed, and they migrate relatively fast. The disorder may occur in infants but is found chiefly in adolescents. It is rare in old people. Acidic food may cause discomfort. The margin may be slightly elevated.

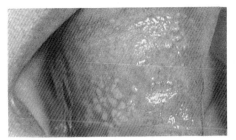

Fig. 381. Heterotopic sebaceous glands

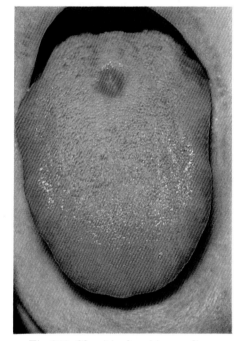

Fig. 382. Glossitis rhombica mediana

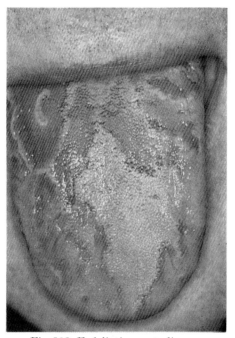

Fig. 383. Exfoliatio areata linguae
(geographic tongue)

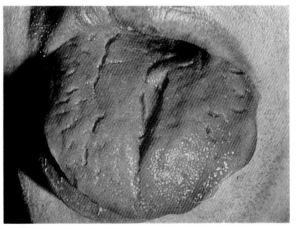

Fig. 384. Scrotal tongue (lingua plicata)

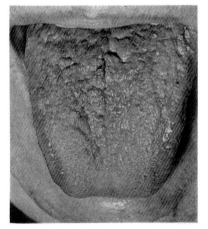

Fig. 385. Black hairy tongue
(lingua nigra)

Lingua plicata

The tongue with indentations and folds, which, if it is severely affected, is called *lingua scrotalis*, presents cerebriform or reticular changes. The furrows often become erosive, rendering acidic or hotly seasoned food painful. Monilia has a special affinity to lingua plicata. The anomaly cannot be considered to be a degenerative stigma, since it has been observed in normal persons. Lingua plicata is one of the signs of the Melkersson-Rosenthal syndrome and may be present in acromegaly. It has been stated that it frequently occurs in patients with psoriasis.

Lingua nigra

The black, hairy tongue presents long and thick bristle-like papillae, chiefly on the medial part of the tongue. Adults develop these changes more frequently than children. The etiology is not always clear. The hyperkeratosis of the filiform papillae may be caused by infections or irritating contacts (for example, oral preparations containing ratanhia). Lately, these changes of the tongue have been observed in patients with disturbed vitamin B metabolism of the gastrointestinal tract following administration of antibiotics.

Fusospirochetosis

The clinical picture of Plaut-Vincent's disease was described as "angina necrotica" by STRÜMPEL in 1883. Although the disease is only slightly contagious, it sometimes appears in epidemic form in adolescents, chiefly in males. In any case, the affected persons do possess teeth. The eruption typically affects one side only, at least in the beginning. General signs are mild, for example, slight enlargement of the regional lymph nodes. Fetor ex ore is pronounced. Grayish-green, diphtheroid pseudomembranes or deep ulcerative changes occur on the tonsils but also on other parts of the oral cavity such as the gingiva of the posterior lower molars. Sometimes bacteriologic evidence of the symbiosis between spirochetes and long fusobacteria is difficult to obtain.

Recurrent or habitual aphthae

Aphthous stomatitis as a first manifestation of an infection by the herpes simplex virus was discussed in connection with viral diseases. The *habitual* or *recurrent aphthae*, described by von MIKULICZ and FLUSSER, are tender and may occur in families. They recur at irregular intervals, rarely with more than two or three lesions. Children are infrequently affected. Victims of the disease are primarily adolescents. Pronounced stomatitis, fetor, and increased salivation are absent.

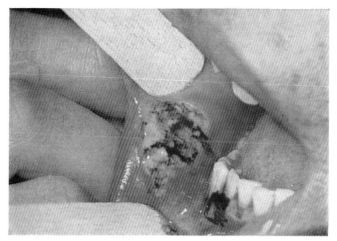

Fig. 386. Plaut -Vincent's stomatitis

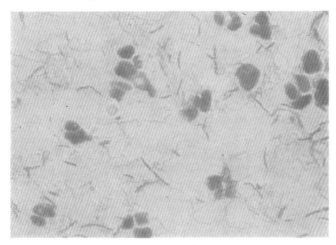

Fig. 387. Plaut -Vincent's fusospirochetosis

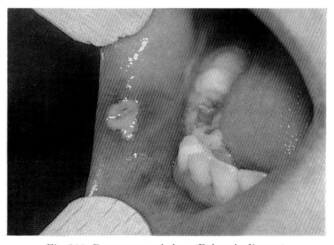

Fig. 388. Recurrent aphthae (Behcet's disease)

31. Venereal Diseases

Of the four venereal diseases only syphilis and gonorrhea are of great importance. There has been an increase of these two conditions in the last eight years, and there has been a definite shift toward the 14 to 18 year age group. A rectal primary syphilitic lesion or primary rectal gonorrhea as a result of homosexual exposure are seen occasionally.* But as far as can be ascertained, the increase of early syphilis seen since 1945 has not resulted in an increase of late syphilis (FROMM and KLUG), and the number of deaths due to late syphilis has actually decreased.

Syphilis

The causative organism of syphilis is the Treponema pallidum discovered on March 3, 1905 by FRITZ SCHAUDINN jointly with E. HOFFMANN. PARACELSUS (1493–1541) had already mentioned coitus, tactus (physical touch), and partus (childbirth) as transmitting the infection. RICORD (1800–1889) recognized the various developmental stages. The primary lesion (an erosive-ulcerated and usually solitary lesion on the skin or mucous membrane, followed shortly by a hard nontender swelling of the regional lymph nodes) appears three weeks after infection. In the secondary stage of acquired syphilis, around the sixth to ninth week after infection, hematogenous generalization of the causative organism takes place. This results first in the appearance of somewhat polymorphic, chiefly macular or papular exanthems, followed later by successively larger but fewer lesions (roséole en retour). Other signs involve the scalp (alopecia diffusa, alopecia areolaris or moth-eaten alopecia) or face, the signe d'omnibus.**

---

* These are rather prevalent in the large cities of the United States. *The translators.*

** An expression of the French school of dermatology, describing how loss of the lateral part of the eyebrows of a passenger riding in a bus permits an observer to make a diagnosis of secondary syphilis. *The translators.*

The oral mucous membranes present mucous patches, chiefly in the form of a specific tonsillitis. Various internal organs such as the liver and kidneys, the muscles, and also the cerebrospinal fluid may be affected. In the tertiary stage, beginning around the fourth or fifth year after infection, a few asymmetrically localized destructive lesions appear, superficially and increasing in size through contact with other lesions (tuberoserpiginous syphilids) or as gummatous syphilomas, which originate in the deep cutis and form hard nodes, which melt slowly.

Syphilis of the child is only seldom acquired ("syphilis of the innocent"). In such rare instances the extragenital primary lesion occurs on the face or the fingers. However, practically all cases of syphilis in children are congenital and result from diaplacental transmission of the treponemes to the fetus ("Without an infected mother there is no syphilitic child," MATZENAUER, 1903). (Rarely, syphilis is acquired intra partum, while the child passes through the birth canal of a mother who has fresh syphilitic lesions acquired in late pregnancy. *The translators*.) In congenital syphilis a true primary lesion per se is missing. The infection is similar to transfusion syphilis or "syphilis d'emblée." Congenital syphilis progresses as a generalized infection; it is rarely evident before the fourth or fifth month of gestation. KASSOWITZ established the rule that the more florid the syphilis of the mother, the earlier the fetus will become infected. Third generation syphilis has been described but seems to be extremely rare. Signs of congenital syphilis differ in the newborn, in infancy, and in the school age child (syphilis congenita tarda). The syphilitic newborn shows facial discoloration of a dirty brown or waxy-white hue (FINKELSTEIN describes the color as that of light milky coffee, TROUSSEAU as that of tobacco stained fingers). There are small or large macular lesions of the skin, similar to the secondary stage of acquired syphilis, a specific coryza (rhinitis), palmoplantar bullae, and pemphigoid lesions with an abundance of spirochetes, present at birth or up to the fourth week. Ulcerations of the navel are rare. At birth maculopapular lesions are seen predominantly on the face and extremities, less frequently on the trunk. Later, perioral scars *(Parrot's rhagades)* permit a diagnosis of congenital syphilis. Circumscribed lesions, such as condylomata lata, occur in the infant. In later life when only a few cutaneous manifestations are present, *Hutchinson's triad* is the main sign. Its manifestations are diffuse interstitial keratitis, pear-shaped and notched upper incisors of the second dentition (PASINI found Treponema pallidum in these teeth), and labyrinth type deafness. The syphilitic infant shows osseous changes such as osteochondritis dissecans (WEGENER, 1870), periostitis syphilitica (sabre shins), and less frequently osteomyelitis fibrosa rareficans (PICK). WEGENER's osteochondritis may be responsible for Parrot's pseudoparalysis of the extremities; in infants, involvement of the joints is the exception. In older children and adolescents, however, the signs of congenital syphilis are saddle nose, frontal or parietal bosses ("front olympique," FOURNIER), and palpable antecubital lymph nodes. Further diagnostic clues are the "tennis racket thumbs" (RONCHESE), the fifth finger sign (DU BOIS), thickening of the sternoclavicular joint (HIGOUMINAKIS), or a chronic enlargement of the salivary glands (NABARRO). Many signs and symptoms (even nocturnal enuresis) formerly ascribed to congenital syphilis are no longer considered to be so. Some mild osseous changes mistakenly called syphilitic were in reality phenocopies caused by the formerly used antisyphilitic drug bismuth. Hemorrhagic phenomena in congenital syphilis are rather complex: a drop in platelets, specific vascular changes, and coagulopathic or paraproteinemic deviations (macroglobulins). Additional noncutaneous signs of congenital syphilis are hepatosplenomegaly (with barely noticeable general lymphadenopathy), macrohematuria due to specific kidney involvement (including hematuria caused by a Herxheimer reaction after the start of syphilitic therapy), interstitial pneumonia, specific neuropathies, and ocular changes (pepper and salt fundus due to syphilitic chorioretinitis; toxoplasmosis must be ruled out).

Serology of syphilis in childhood

In the absence of syphilitic manifestations it is sometimes necessary to perform several classic serologic tests and to weigh their results in order to decide whether syphilis is present.

A newborn child with positive results to all or a few serologic tests may actually suffer from congenital syphilis (in most instances there are also clinical signs), or a transfer of antibodies or reagins from mother to child might have occurred. The antibodies or reagins usually disappear from the serum after a period of about three to six months. Older infants or young children might show nonspecific positive reactions (see TPI test below).

Should the serologic reactions in a newborn infant be negative, it still has to be proved that the child is free from syphilis. The child might be in the incubation period when serologic tests are still negative, or the positive serology of the unborn child in utero might have reverted back to negative because of antisyphilitic treatment of the mother during pregnancy. In such circumstances the syphilis of the mother has either been cured or has entered a seronegative latent period.

Small children with untreated congenital syphilis usually have positive serologic tests; only at a later age do these children enter a seronegative latent period.

Serologic results in older children have to be evaluated as those of adults.

A positive *Treponema Immobilization Test (TPI)* of Nelson in a newborn child without clinical manifestations of syphilis does not prove the child has syphilis, because of the presence of maternal immobilizing antibodies in the blood of the child; the antibodies usually disappear from the serum after three to six months.

A decision as to the absence of a syphilitic infection in the child is facilitated if the titer of the infant's serum is significantly lower than that of the mother (and if, on further testing every few weeks, the titer keeps dropping. *The translators*).

A negative TPI (NELSON) test at birth does not disprove the presence of syphilis because this test may become positive later. Therefore, the decision as to an intrauterine infection cannot rest upon the TPI test of the newborn or small infant.

In later childhood the TPI test (or the more recent Fluorescent Treponema Antibody [FTA-ABS] test, which is simpler and less expensive. *The translators*) is positive if syphilis is present. If negative, it can be used to invalidate nonspecific positive classic serologic reactions.

As a rule, antisyphilitic treatment of the child results in seronegativity the earlier the treatment has been started.

Gonorrhea

The causative organism of gonorrhea was discovered in 1879 by the then 23 year old ALBERT NEISSER, and was called "gonococcus" by his classmate PAUL EHRLICH. Today it is called Neisseria gonorrhoeae. Other organisms belonging to the Neisseria group are the meningococcus and Neisseria catarrhalis. This "form of micrococcus specific for gonorrhea" (NEISSER) is gram-negative; so, however, are all pseudogonococci. A few days after an infection the organisms stained with methylene blue represent coffee bean-shaped diplococci, arranged (through phagocytosis) like a swarm of bees within a cell. They are all of the same size (0.6 to 1.0 micron). In legal cases culture plates inoculated with the pus are imperative. After a short incubation period of one to eight days the male shows urethral discharge. The female shows urethral and cervical involvement. Sometimes the vaginal secretion contaminates the rectum, causing gonorrheic proctitis.

This highly infectious disease does not confer immunity. In the female child the vagina itself becomes infected ("vulvovaginitis gonorrheica"). Whereas the squamous vaginal epithelium of the sexually mature woman is immune to gonorrheic infection, the ischemic genital tract of the senile woman behaves like the vagina of the child. Vulvovaginitis gonorrheica infantum, transmitted by means of sponges, wet towels, and so forth, can easily be overlooked

216

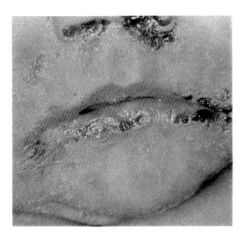

Fig. 389. Congenital syphilis (coryza).
Beginning Parrot's rhagades.

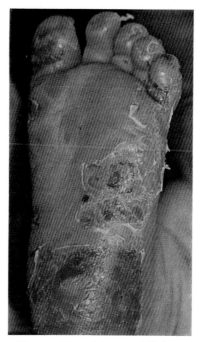

Fig. 390. Pemphigus syphiliticus

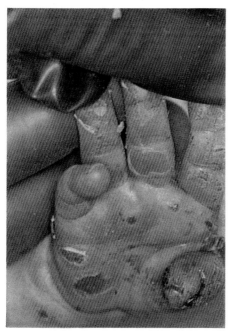

Fig. 391. Pemphigus syphiliticus

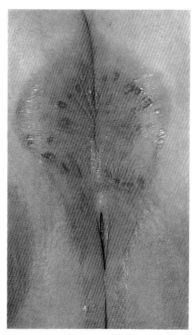

Fig. 392. Condylomata lata

217

in children who bathe frequently, because of a lack of signs.* Other children present a rather stormy course, with urinary difficulties and profuse purulent secretion behind the hymenal opening, causing yellowish green spots on the underwear. Differential diagnosis includes consideration of intestinal parasites, oxyuriasis, trichomoniasis, and others.

Gonorrheic vulvovaginitis is rarely followed by a *gonorrheic infection of the eye*. Sometimes accidental contamination with pus from an adult causes usually unilateral ocular infection. In the newborn a bilateral infection of the eyes can be acquired while the child passes through the genital tract. At first catarrhal inflammation and infiltration are present, leading then to blenorrhea neonatorum proper with its characteristic grayish-yellow secretion of pus from the space between the swollen eyelids. Gonorrheic infection of the eye in the adult is more dangerous because resulting corneal ulcers may lead to blindness. The cornea of the newborn seems to offer more resistance (PILLAT).

---

* Vulvovaginitis may also be transmitted through direct contact with the mother if the child sleeps in the same bed.

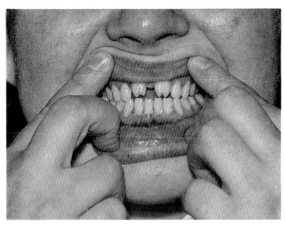

Fig. 393. Late manifestation of congenital syphilis. Hutchinson's teeth.

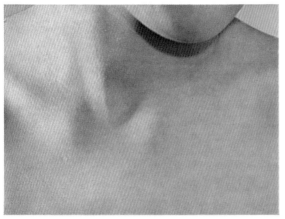

Fig. 394. Late manifestation of congenital syphilis. Periosteal swelling of the sternal end of clavicle. (Clavicular sign of Higouménakis)

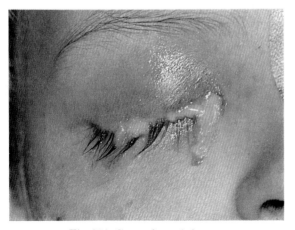

Fig. 396. Gonorrhea of the eye

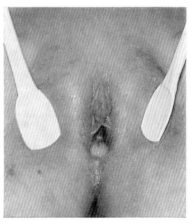

Fig. 395. Gonorrheic vulvovaginitis of little girls

32. Nonvenereal Diseases of the Genitals

Balanitis

The terms balanitis and balanoposthitis describe superficial inflammations of the glans penis or the glans penis and prepuce. They present different clinical pictures and etiology. *Balanitis of small boys* is similar to "seborrheic" balanitis and is caused by the constant irritation of secretions and mechanical insults aggravated by microbial infections. Secondary balanitis is observed in boys with elongated (elephant's trunk-like) foreskins (phimosis) and concomitant impaired urination.

Boys up to the first year of life may show physiologic adherence of the inner prepuce to the glans penis. The two become separated, however, when smegma is produced. If the separation does not take place, a pathologic condition ensues. Another cause of phimosis is a congenital stenosis of the preputial ring.

While Reiter's disease (1916) is primarily a condition of adult males, it may occur occasionally in children. The triad of arthritis, conjunctivitis, and urethritis is sometimes accompanied by "balanitis circinata parakeratotica" (REICH), also known as Reiter's balanitis, with delicate grayish-white, psoriasiform-keratotic lesions or moist macules with a thin, scaly border.

Although diphtheria has become a rarity, the even rarer *balanitis diphtherica* is usually observed in childhood as a secondary manifestation. Diphtheria of the genital tract was formerly more frequent in girls than in boys. Belanitis erosiva circinata and balanoposthitis plasmacellularis are seen only in adults.

Ulcus vulvae acutum

Lipschütz's and Scherber's ulcus vulvae acutum* occasionally presents a hyperacute condition with impressive systemic signs (HAMMERSCHMIDT and KORTING: primary atypical pneumonia with increased cold agglutinins). The condition should be called vulvitis aphthosa (in analogy to stomatitis aphthosa). The first attack of this disease affects 14 to 20 year old girls (LIPSCHÜTZ), mostly virgins. Recurrences are the rule. Occasionally, changes of the oral mucosa or a "specific" erythema nodosum may accompany or alternate with the vulval lesion. LIPSCHÜTZ thought that Döderlein's bacillus found in the genital lesions was the etiologic agent, but its presence is now considered to be coincidental. The lesions vary in size from miliary to gangrenous ulcers causing severe pain on urination.

---

* Many authors consider ulcus vulvae acutum a manifestation of Behcet's syndrome or Touraine's "grande aphthose." *(The translators)*.

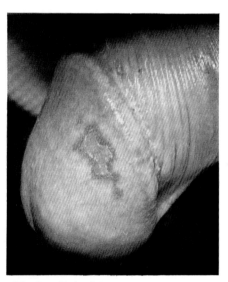

Fig. 397. Balanitis circinata parakeratotica in Reiter's disease

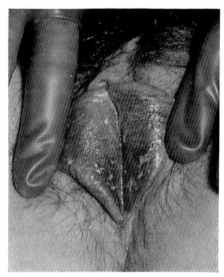

Fig. 398. Multiple lesions of ulcus vulvae
acutum or vulvitis aphthosa
(Behcet's disease)

Index

Page numbers in *italics* indicate illustrations.